T5-DIA-703

LIBRARY/NEW ENGLAND INST. OF TECHNOLOGY
3 0147 1003 9299 5

WHAT'S A [...] TO DO

A Collection of OT Activities

Felicia Norman, COTA

Therapy
Skill Builders®
a division of
The Psychological Corporation
555 Academic Court
San Antonio, Texas 78204-2498
1-800-228-0752

Reproducing Pages From This Book

As described below, some of the pages in this book may be reproduced for instructional use (not for resale). To protect your book, make a photocopy of each reproducible page. Then use that copy as a master for photocopying.

Therapy Skill Builders® ®
a division of
The Psychological Corporation
555 Academic Court
San Antonio, Texas 78204-2498
1-800-228-0752

Printed in the United States of America

ISBN 0761634002

2 3 4 5 6 7 8 9 10 11 12 A B C D E

Visit our website at www.hbtpc.com

Preface

"We need you to run a group," is a statement that strikes fear in most health care professionals. It was also the impetus for creating *What's a Group to Do?,* a collection of activities put together to make the task of running a group easier for health care professionals and more therapeutic for the participants.

What's a Group to Do? is designed to be used by any Occupational, Physical, or Recreational Therapist; or Speech Language Pathologist, with participants varying in age and functional abilities.

Each activity includes *Required Function Levels* information so that you can see at a glance what cognitive, sensorimotor, and interpersonal skill levels participants must have.

What's a Group to Do? Have fun! So, go have fun with your group!

About the Author

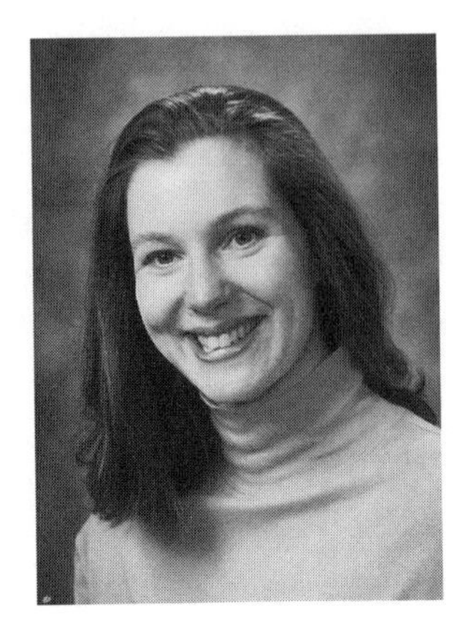

Felicia Norman completed the occupational therapy assistant program at Grand Rapids Community College in Michigan and received her certification in California. Ms. Norman began developing her repertoire of group activities as an intern, working with children with disabilities in school settings and adults in a variety of rehab settings. She has worked with geriatric, neurological, and orthopedic patients in retraining activities of daily living, cognitive skills, improving range of motion, and strengthening exercises through group activities and individual therapy.

Table of Contents

Crafts

Appendix

introduction

The purpose of these group activities is to improve the participants' entry level of function. Function levels, for the purpose of this book, are identified *assessed* levels of function. As the group leader, you need to make sure that a qualified professional has determined each participant's function level to ensure that the activity is appropriate and safe.

General Therapeutic Goals and Objectives are listed at the beginning of each section of activities. They are listed in order of significance. The goals listed are comprehensive, but may not be all inclusive. Each group activity includes a list of Therapeutic Goals. You may choose to modify the goals or create new ones as is appropriate to the activity and the participants' function levels.

Like function levels, receptive and expressive communication are important components of the *group process.* Each activity has been organized to encourage interaction between participants, both during and following the group activity. It is up to you as the leader to facilitate and monitor appropriate communication to ensure its therapeutic value.

Definitions of Function Levels

Cognitive Skills

Cognitive skills are the abilities to manage or process events (e.g., problem-solving and planning). Skill components may involve *orientation, memory, attention span, conceptualization, judgment,* and *communication.*

Skill level ratings

3 Group is appropriate for individuals with **minimal or no limitations** in this area. Participant must be able to follow moderately complex verbal instructions, *attend to the task for more than 30 minutes,* complete multi-step tasks with minimal verbal or visual cues, and communicate effectively orally.

2 Group is appropriate for individuals with **moderate limitations** in this area. Participant must be able to follow simple verbal instructions, *attend to the task for 15 to 30 minutes,* complete tasks of three steps or less with moderate verbal or visual cues, and communicate effectively orally or with gestures.

1 Group is appropriate for individuals with **severe limitations** in this area. Participant must be able to follow either very simple verbal instructions or demonstration, *attend to the task for less than 15 minutes,* complete 1- to 2-step tasks with maximum verbal cues and physical assistance, and communicate orally or with gestures.

Sensorimotor Skills

Sensorimotor skills are the abilities to receive and interpret sensory information and to affect motor responses. Skill components include *range of motion, muscle strength, muscle tone, endurance, fine motor skills, and visual and auditory acuity/perception.*

Skill level ratings

3 Group is appropriate for individuals with **minimal or no limitations.** Participant is able to safely and effectively manipulate self and objects *independently or with minimal assistance* with or without assistive devices, or *require visual supervision.*

2 Group is appropriate for individuals with **minimal to moderate limitations** in this area. Participant requires *minimal to moderate physical assistance,* or standby/contact guard to safely and effectively manipulate self and objects.

1 Group is appropriate for individuals with **moderate to severe limitations** in this area. Participant requires *moderate to maximum assistance* to manipulate self and objects safely and effectively.

Interpersonal Skills

Interpersonal skills are the abilities to coordinate/regulate one's own behavior to effectively interact with others to meet mutual needs or accomplish mutual activities and goals in a group setting.

Skill level ratings

3 Group is appropriate for individuals with **minimal or no limitations.** Participant is able to work with others beyond the needs of the specific task, to work cooperatively to complete relatively long-range activities, and fairly consistently demonstrates respect for the rights of others.

2 Group is appropriate for individuals with **moderate limitations.** Participant requires moderate assistance to become involved in group for a short-term task that requires sharing/interaction.

1 Group is appropriate for individuals with **severe limitations.** Participant's interaction is limited to minimal sharing of the task.

COOKING ACTIVITIES

Toast With Butter

No-Bake Cookies

Healthy Dip

Marshmallow Cereal Cookies

Cereal Fries

Frozen Fruit Fun

Note: In choosing activities from the following section, it is important that you consider age, safety awareness, and the appropriateness of an activity based on each participant's evaluated function level. As the leader of the group, you are responsible for ensuring that all health and safety precautions are followed during the group activity. For all cooking activities, you should have on hand

* measuring spoons
* mixing/stirring spoons
* measuring cup(s) (preferably plastic)
* paper towels
* newspapers

Sample Measurable Objectives for Cooking Activities

Goal: To increase or maintain range of motion.
Objective: Patient's range of motion in *(specify upper extremity joint[s])* will be maintained or increased *(specify degrees or functional limits).*

Goal: To increase or maintain strength and endurance.
Objective: Patient will increase or maintain overall muscle strength and endurance.
Objective: Patient will increase or maintain muscle strength and endurance in *(specify specific muscle group[s] or extremities).*

Goal: To increase or maintain ability to attend to the task.
Objective: Patient will attend to the activity for *(specify length of time).*
Objective: Patient will attend to the group for *(specify length of time).*

Goal: To improve socialization skills.
Objective: Patient will be able to work on an activity without disrupting others in the group.
Objective: Patient will work cooperatively on activity with another patient or others.

Goal: To improve or maintain receptive communication skills.
Objective: Patient will be able to follow a simple demonstration.
Objective: Patient will be able to follow one-step oral directions.
Objective: Patient will be able to follow multi-step oral directions.

Goal: To improve or maintain expressive communication skills.
Objective: Patient will use gestures to indicate needs.
Objective: Patient will use single words verbally to express needs.
Objective: Patient will use phrases or sentences verbally to express needs.

Toast With Butter

This is a good mid-morning activity!

Required Function Levels

Cognitive: 3–2
Sensorimotor: 3–2
Interpersonal: 3–1

Group Size 3–10

Materials

2 or more pints of heavy whipping cream (depending on size of group)
1 small empty plastic container with a lid or 1 baby food jar with a lid for each participant
Toast (enough for group)
Jam
Plastic knives
Newspapers

Directions

Have participants

1. spread newspaper out on the floor or on the table where they will sit or stand
2. wash their hands and keep the area clean during the activity
3. sit or stand at their areas
4. measure 1 tablespoon of whipping cream into each container. (A higher functioning client might be able to assist in measuring out whipping cream into plastic containers and dispersing them among the group.)
5. secure the lid on the container
6. shake the container until a lump of butter forms (about 7 minutes)
7. use the plastic knife to remove butter from the jar and spread on toast
8. spread jam on top of the buttered toast

Therapeutic Goals

1. To increase or maintain current range of motion.
2. To increase or maintain endurance.
3. To increase or maintain strength.
4. To increase or maintain ability to attend to the task.
5. To increase or maintain ability to complete the task.
6. To improve socialization skills.
7. To improve or maintain receptive communication skills.
8. To improve or maintain expressive communication skills.

Contraindications Dietary restrictions

Variations Participant(s) might request assistance for balance if he or she is standing.

Comments and Observations

No-Bake Cookies

Required Function Levels

Cognitive: 3–2
Sensorimotor: 3–2
Interpersonal: 3–1

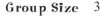

Group Size 3–5

Materials

1/2 C. peanut butter
1/3 C. honey
1/2 C. coconut flakes
2 1/2 C. cereal (crunchy oats type and/or crispy rice type for texture)
Extras: raisins, dates, banana chips, chocolate chips
Large bowl
Cookie tray
Wax paper
Large mixing spoon
Paper towels

Directions

Have participants sit around a table. Each will be in charge of measuring and adding an ingredient to the mixing bowl. Have participants take turns stirring the ingredients and dropping mixture by the spoonful onto the cookie tray. Instruct everyone to wash their hands and keep the area clean during the activity.

1. Divide the tasks of measuring, adding, and mixing ingredients among participants.
2. Set aside the bowl, peanut butter, honey, coconut, and extras.
3. Have participants add ingredients to the bowl and mix well.
4. Stir in 1/2 C. of the cereal.
5. Place the remaining 2 C. of cereal in another bowl.
6. Shape spoonfuls of the peanut butter mixture into balls.
7. Roll peanut butter balls in the extra cereal.
8. Place cookies on a cookie tray.
9. Chill cookies in refrigerator for 15–20 minutes before eating.

Therapeutic Goals

1. To increase or maintain range of motion.
2. To increase or maintain strength and coordination in upper extremities.
3. To increase or maintain strength and endurance.
4. To increase or maintain ability to attend to the task.
5. To increase or maintain ability to complete the task.
6. To increase or maintain ability to follow directions.
7. To improve socialization skills.
8. To improve or maintain receptive communication skills.
9. To improve or maintain expressive communication skills.

Contraindications

Dietary restrictions
Impulsiveness—eating while performing group activity may spread germs.

Comments and Observations

Healthy Dip

Required Function Levels
Cognitive: 3–2
Sensorimotor: 3–2
Interpersonal: 3–2

Group Size 3–8

Materials
1/2 C. cottage cheese (nonfat or low fat)
1/4 C. grated cheddar cheese
2 tsp. dill weed or parsley
1 tsp. Worcestershire sauce
Pinch of salt
Assorted vegetables (precut and cleaned would be easiest)
Mixing bowl
Spoon for mixing

Directions Instruct everyone to wash their hands and keep the area clean during the activity. Have participants sit around a table. Each one will be in charge of measuring and adding an ingredient to the mixing bowl or cleaning vegetables.

1. Assign the tasks of measuring and adding ingredients among group participants.
2. Have the participants measure and add the cottage cheese, grated cheese, dill or parsley, Worcestershire sauce, and salt into the mixing bowl.
3. Mix together until blended.
4. Clean and prepare vegetables for eating.
5. Dip the vegetables and enjoy!

Therapeutic Goals

1. To increase or maintain range of motion.
2. To increase or maintain strength and coordination in upper extremities.
3. To increase or maintain strength and endurance.
4. To increase or maintain ability to attend to the task.
5. To increase or maintain ability to complete the task.
6. To increase or maintain ability to follow directions.
7. To improve or maintain receptive communication skills.
8. To improve or maintain expressive communication skills.
9. To improve socialization skills.
10. To provide tactile, gustatory, and olfactory stimulation.

Contraindications
Dietary restrictions
Impulsiveness—eating while handling ingredients (i.e., sticking fingers in the mixture) may spread germs.

Comments and Observations

Marshmallow Cereal Cookies

Required Function Levels

Cognitive: 3–2
Sensorimotor: 3–2
Interpersonal: 3–2

Group Size 3–5

Materials

5 C. marshmallows
1/2 C. butter
3 C. (or more) of cereal (crispy rice type, or several different kinds)
Deep saucepan
Wooden spoons
Wax paper

Directions

Instruct everyone to wash their hands and keep the area clean during the activity. Some standing is required for melting the ingredients, although it may be possible to perform from wheelchair level if stove is accessible. Each participant will be in charge of measuring and adding an ingredient.

1. Divide these tasks among group participants.
2. Place marshmallows and butter in saucepan.
3. Place saucepan over low heat to melt ingredients. Stir until blended.
4. Let mixture cool.
5. Stir cereal into the mixture until it is thoroughly coated.
6. Have participants shape spoonfuls of the mixture into balls.
7. After they have shaped the mixture in balls, have participants place them on wax paper to cool.

Therapeutic Goals

1. To increase or maintain range of motion.
2. To increase or maintain strength and coordination in upper extremities.
3. To increase or maintain strength and endurance.
4. To increase or maintain ability to attend to the task.
5. To increase or maintain ability to complete the task.
6. To increase or maintain ability to follow directions.
7. To improve or maintain receptive communication skills.
8. To improve or maintain expressive communication skills.
9. To provide tactile, gustatory, and olfactory stimulation.
10. To improve or maintain socialization skills.

Contraindications

Dietary restrictions
Impulsiveness—no eating on the job!

Comments and Observations

Cereal Fries

Required Function Levels

Cognitive: 3–2
Sensorimotor: 3–2
Interpersonal: 3–2

Group Size 3–5

Materials
- 2/3 C. grated cheese
- 1/4 C. soft butter
- 1/3 C. + 2 tsp. flour
- 1/3 C. + 2 tsp. crispy rice-type cereal
- Bowl
- Pastry cutter
- Cookie tray
- Spoon

Directions Instruct everyone to wash their hands and maintain a clean environment during the activity. Some standing is required for getting tray in and out of oven, although it may be possible to perform from wheelchair level if oven is accessible. Each participant will be in charge of measuring and adding an ingredient.

1. Place butter, flour, cereal, and grated cheese in the bowl.
2. Divide these tasks among members in the group.
3. Stir well until thoroughly blended.
4. Form dough into balls and place on a cookie tray.
5. Bake at 375° for 10 minutes.
6. Allow to cool before eating.

Therapeutic Goals

1. To increase or maintain range of motion.
2. To increase or maintain strength and coordination in upper extremities.
3. To increase or maintain strength and endurance.
4. To increase or maintain ability to attend to task.
5. To increase or maintain ability to complete the task.
6. To increase or maintain ability to follow directions.
7. To improve or maintain receptive communication skills.
8. To improve or maintain expressive communication skills.
9. To provide tactile, gustatory, and olfactory stimulation.
10. To improve or maintain socialization skills.

Contraindications Dietary restrictions

Comments and Observations

Frozen Fruit Fun

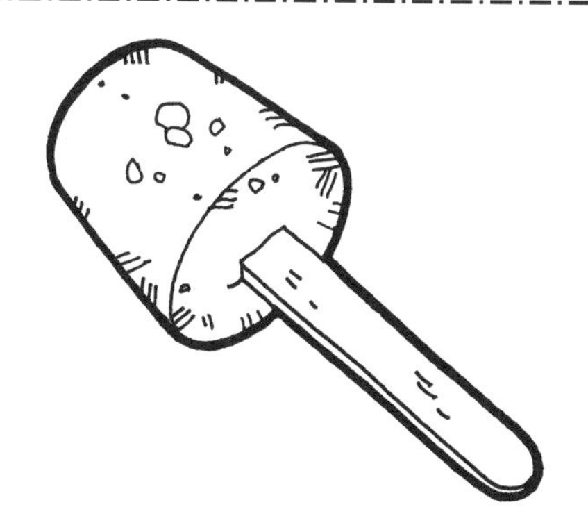

Members of the group will need to use their imaginations for concocting the *perfect frozen fruit.* Make enough to share with the other people in the facility or have a taste contest. Who made the best one? Fun summer activity or in the middle of winter, turn up the heat in the therapy room to do this.

Required Function Levels

Cognitive: 3–2
Sensorimotor: 3–2
Interpersonal: 3–2

Group Size 3–5

Materials

Craft sticks or small plastic spoons
Small mixing bowls
Small paper cups
Things to use in the frozen mixture: fruit juice, yogurt, chocolate milk, breakfast mix, fruit

Directions

Instruct everyone to wash their hands and keep the area clean during the activity.

1. Have participants decide what materials they want to use (yogurt, breakfast mix with a little fruit juice and small pieces of fruit).
2. In a bowl, have each member mix their own concoction.
3. Have each person write his or her name on outside of the paper cups he or she is using.
4. Have each person pour mixture into paper cup, about 2/3 full.
5. Stick in freezer.
6. When mixture starts to freeze, insert sticks or spoons.
7. Return the cups to the freezer and allow to freeze completely.
8. Eat when frozen!

Therapeutic Goals

1. To increase or maintain range of motion.
2. To increase or maintain strength and coordination in upper extremities.
3. To increase or maintain strength and endurance.
4. To increase or maintain ability to attend to the task.
5. To increase or maintain ability to complete the task.
6. To increase or maintain ability to follow directions.
7. To improve or maintain receptive communication skills.
8. To improve or maintain expressive communication skills.
9. To provide tactile, gustatory, and olfactory stimulation.
10. To improve or maintain socialization skills.

Contraindications Dietary restrictions

Comments and Observations

Gross Motor Activities

Foam Faces

Macaroni Maracas

Bell Bracelets

Marching to Music

Long Shot

Stop and Go

Mimic the Leader

Wishing Well

Crazy Walk

Ladybug, Ladybug Fly Away

Note: In choosing activities from the following section, it is important that you consider age, safety awareness, and appropriateness of an activity based on each participant's evaluated function level. As the leader of the group, you are responsible for ensuring that all health and safety precautions are followed during the group activity.

Sample Measurable Objectives for Gross Motor Activities

Goal: To increase or maintain range of motion.

Objective: Patients' range of motion in *(specify upper extremity joint[s])* will be maintained or increased *(specify degrees or within functional limits).*

Goal: To increase or maintain strength and endurance.

Objective: Patient will increase or maintain overall muscle strength and endurance.

Objective: Patient will increase or maintain muscle strength and endurance in *(specify specific muscle group[s] or extremities).*

Goal: To increase or maintain balance.

Objective: Patient will increase or maintain ability to stand *(specify length of time)* with an assistive device.

Objective: Patient will increase or maintain ability to stand *(specify length of time)* without an assistive device.

Goal: To increase or maintain ability to attend to the task.

Objective: Patient will attend to the activity for *(specify length of time).*

Objective: Patient will attend to the group for *(specify length of time).*

Goal: To improve socialization skills.

Objective: Patient will be able to work on the activity without disrupting others.

Objective: Patient will work cooperatively on the activity with another patient or others.

Goal: To improve or maintain receptive communication skills.

Objective: Patient will be able to follow a simple demonstration.

Objective: Patient will be able to follow one-step oral directions.

Objective: Patient will be able to follow multi-step oral directions.

Goal: To improve or maintain expressive communication skills.

Objective: Patient will use gestures to indicate needs.

Objective: Patient will use single words verbally to express needs.

Objective: Patient will use phrases or sentences verbally to express needs.

Goal: To provide tactile stimulation.

Objective: Patient will be able to identify objects on the basis of touch.

Objective: Patient will discriminate between objects on the basis of texture.

Goal: To increase or maintain fine motor skills.

Objective: Patient will demonstrate fine motor dexterity *(specify unilateral or bilateral).*

Goal: To provide olfactory stimulation.

Objective: Patient will be able to identify objects on the basis of smell.

Foam Faces

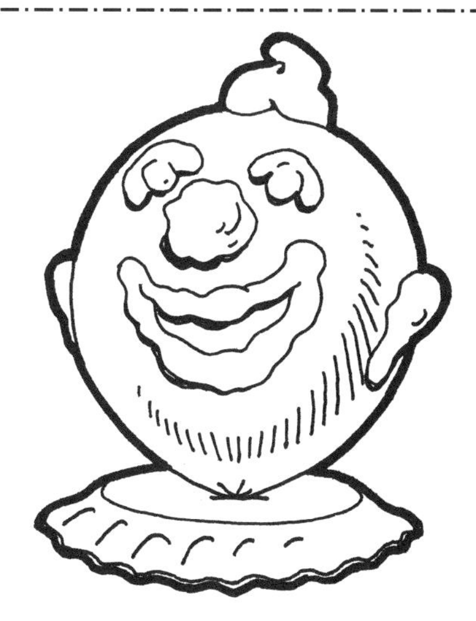

Required Function Levels

Cognitive: 3–2
Sensorimotor: 3–2
Interpersonal: 3–1

Group Size 4–8, depending on seating availability

Materials
2–4 cans of shaving cream
Balloons
Paper plates
Scissors

Directions Have participants sit around a table to work on this project.

1. Cut a slit in the middle of each paper plate (or have the patients do it) and use as a base for the balloon.
2. Inflate a balloon for each client, or have the patient do it if he or she is able.
3. Have the patients push the knotted end of the balloon through the slit in the plate and set it on the table.
4. Distribute cans of shaving cream, 1 can per participant.
5. Have each person shake the can of shaving cream before using it. You may have the patient shake the can with one hand and then the other, or use both hands at once.
6. Have each person decorate the balloon to make it look like a face.

Therapeutic Goals

1. To increase or maintain range of motion.
2. To increase or maintain fine motor strength and coordination.
3. To increase or maintain strength and endurance.
4. To increase or maintain ability to attend to the task.
5. To increase or maintain ability to complete the task.
6. To improve socialization skills.
7. To improve or maintain receptive communication skills.
8. To improve or maintain expressive communication skills.
9. To improve or maintain creative thinking.
10. To improve or maintain decision-making process.
11. To provide olfactory stimulation.
12. To provide tactile stimulation.

Contraindications Allergy or sensitivity to shaving cream

Variations

* Use silly string for more color and silly designs.
* Use finger paints for color and more intricate designs.

Comments and Observations

Macaroni Maracas

Required Function Levels

Cognitive: 3–2
Sensorimotor: 3–2
Interpersonal: 3–1

Group Size 3–10

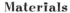

Materials

A room large enough for all participants to stand in, an arm's length apart
A compact disc or cassette player that is loud enough for the participants to hear
Music with appropriate tempos the group can follow/for the skill level of the group
Long necked plastic bottles with caps (e.g., ketchup, relish, chocolate syrup bottles)
Filler material—rice, various beans, birdseed, macaroni
Masking tape
Several colors of yarn or ribbon cut in 12" lengths

Directions

1. Pass bottles out to the participants or have them choose the one they want.
2. Have participants fill their bottles to various levels with filler material.
3. Seal bottles with bottle caps or masking tape.
4. Have participants cut the lengths of yarn or ribbon.
5. Have participants tie lengths of colorful yarn or ribbons to the necks of the bottles for decoration.
6. Have each participant hold the neck of the bottle and shake it to the rhythm of the music.

Have participants shake maracas to music, your clapping, or no sounds at all. Marching is a good activity to create an aerobic workout. This activity may require Restorative Nursing Assistants or Physical Therapists if participants want to stand. This will require group cooperation to get a good beat going, not just noise. Participants may be seated in wheelchairs for this activity.

Therapeutic Goals

1. To increase or maintain range of motion.
2. To increase or maintain strength and coordination in upper extremities.
3. If done with PT, to increase or maintain coordination of both extremities.
4. To increase tactile stimulation, auditory stimulation and discrimination.
5. To increase or maintain strength and endurance.
6. To increase or maintain ability to attend to the task.
7. To increase or maintain ability to complete the task.
8. To increase or maintain ability to follow directions.
9. To improve or maintain receptive communication skills.
10. To improve or maintain expressive communication skills.

Contraindications

Sensitivity to noise
Eating filler materials

Variations

* Use with *Bell Bracelets* from following activity for more auditory stimulation.
* Use maracas in *Marching to Music* activity.

Comments and Observations

Bell Bracelets

Required Function Levels
Cognitive: 3–2
Sensorimotor: 3–2
Interpersonal: 3–1

Group Size 3–8

Materials Narrow ribbon 1/8" to 1/4" wide
(or colored elastic string same width)
Small to medium size bells in a variety of types and colors

Directions Have participants sit around a table. This activity *requires a minimal amount of socialization,* although it may increase, depending on the participants.

1. Cut the ribbon into 6" to 8" lengths.
2. Give each person bells and ribbon to create a bracelet.
3. String bells onto ribbon (about 4 bells per ribbon).
4. Tie knots on each side of the bells to secure placement.
5. Tie the ribbon onto the participant's wrist or, if you're using elastic, knot the two ends together.
6. Encourage full range of motion in arms for a variety of sounds.

Therapeutic Goals

1. To increase or maintain range of motion.
2. To increase or maintain strength and coordination in upper extremities.
3. To increase tactile stimulation, auditory stimulation and discrimination.
4. To increase or maintain strength and endurance.
5. To increase or maintain ability to attend to the task.
6. To increase or maintain ability to complete the task.
7. To increase or maintain fine motor strength and coordination.
8. To increase or maintain ability to follow directions.
9. To improve or maintain receptive communication skills.
10. To improve or maintain expressive communication skills.

Contraindications Sensitivity to noise

Variations

* Use holiday-colored ribbons.
* Jingle to different kinds of music from all over the world.
* Tie the bells on participants' ankles to encourage movement of the entire body.

Comments and Observations

Marching to Music

Required Function Levels
Cognitive: 3–2
Sensorimotor: 3–2
Interpersonal: 3–2

Group Size 3–8

Materials
Floor space
Compact disc or cassette tape player
Compact discs or audiocassette tapes
Items with which to make noise

Directions Have participants stand in a circle or sit in chairs with their feet on the floor to march in place. To march from sitting position, have participants keep their hips and knees in flexion and lift their upper legs off the chair and one foot off the floor, varying this from side to side. Change the beat of the music to stimulate various marching rhythms. Ask members to clap their hands to create the marching beat. Incorporate *Bell Bracelets* and *Macaroni Maracas* to create a different atmosphere.

1. Set a steady pace by clapping your hands and start marching.
2. Introduce *Maracas* to get arms moving and set beat.
3. Slowly increase the pace of marching.
4. Introduce *Bell Bracelets* for variety.
5. Slowly decrease the pace of marching.

Therapeutic Goals

1. To increase or maintain range of motion.
2. To increase or maintain strength and coordination in upper extremities.
3. To stimulate auditory processing and discrimination when following beat.
4. To increase or maintain strength and endurance.
5. To increase or maintain ability to attend to the task.
6. To increase or maintain ability to complete the task.
7. To increase or maintain range of motion, strength, and endurance in lower extremities.
8. To increase or maintain balance.
9. To increase or maintain ability to follow directions.
10. To improve or maintain receptive communication skills.
11. To improve or maintain expressive communication skills.
12. Increase proprioception awareness.

Contraindications Sensitivity to noise

Variations Some old marching songs played on a machine might be fun in a geriatric setting.

Comments and Observations

Long Shot

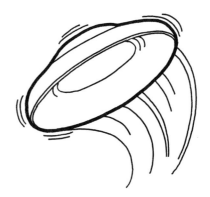

Required Function Levels

Cognitive: 3–2
Sensorimotor: 3–2
Interpersonal: 3–1

Group Size As many eager participants as possible. Organize small groups of 3–5 to start.

Materials

Frisbee®-type flying disk
Craft sticks
Masking tape
Felt pen
Yardstick for base line

Directions This should be played outside where there is ample space or in a gym or hallway. The object is to throw the disk as far as possible and beat any previous records.

1. Have each participant write his or her name on a craft stick.
2. Have the first participant throw the disk from the base line.
3. After disk lands, place the craft stick with the participant's name where the disk landed.
4. Have participants take turns, until everyone has had a chance to throw the disk.
5. If playing in a hallway or gym, use masking tape to secure the craft stick, marking where the disk lands.

Therapeutic Goals

1. To increase or maintain range of motion.
2. To increase or maintain strength and coordination in upper extremities.
3. To increase or maintain strength and endurance.
4. To increase or maintain balance.
5. To increase or maintain ability to attend to the task.
6. To increase or maintain ability to complete the task.
7. To increase or maintain ability to follow directions.
8. To improve or maintain receptive communication skills.
9. To improve or maintain expressive communication skills.

Comments and Observations

Stop and Go

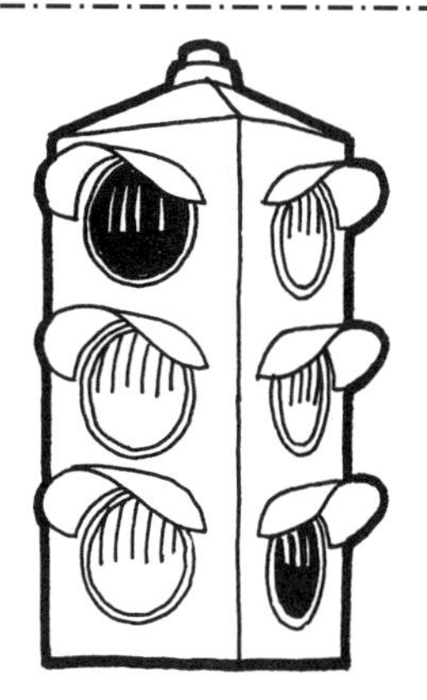

Required Function Levels

Cognitive: 3–2
Sensorimotor: 3–2
Interpersonal: 3–1

Group Size 3–10

Materials None

Directions Choose a leader to be the one who starts and stops the group by clapping. Participants will move around room in wheelchair or by walking until leader claps hands and says "stop." The participants should stop and not move until the leader claps and says "go." Encourage participants to use full range of motion when moving their arms, hands, feet, neck, head—*all parts of their bodies!*

1. Have participants move about room, using full range of motion in all joints.
2. Leader will clap hands and say "stop."
3. Everyone should "stop" in their tracks.
4. See how long participants can stay motionless.
5. Leader will clap hands and say "go."
6. Participants can start ranging joints again.

Therapeutic Goals

1. To increase or maintain range of motion.
2. To increase or maintain strength and coordination in upper extremities.
3. To increase or maintain strength and endurance.
4. To increase or maintain balance.
5. To increase or maintain ability to attend to the task.
6. To increase or maintain ability to complete the task.
7. To increase or maintain ability to follow directions.
8. To improve or maintain receptive communication skills.
9. To improve or maintain expressive communication skills.
10. To increase or maintain strength and coordination of lower extremities.

Variations

* Have the leader use a whistle instead of clapping; participants will hear it better.
* Each time the leader says "go," tell the participants to focus on range of motion for one area (e.g., hands and wrists, elbows, shoulders).
* After the leader says "stop," he or she can call out an activity to be done (e.g., neck circles and nods, rocking back and forth on balls of feet) while participants are stopped.
* Flick lights on and off for participants who are hearing impaired.

Comments and Observations

Mimic the Leader

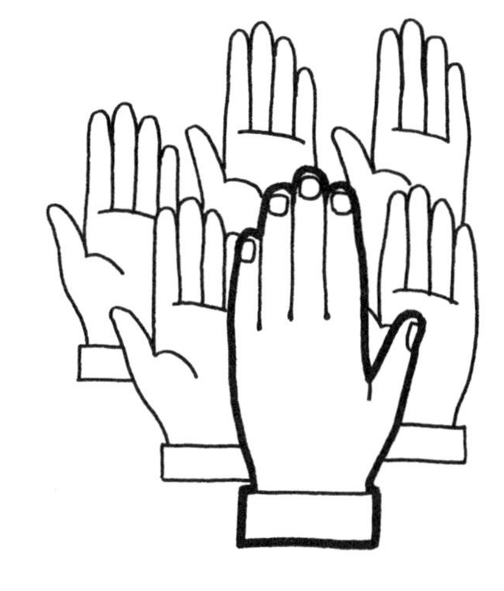

Required Function Levels
Cognitive: 3–2
Sensorimotor: 3–2
Interpersonal: 3–1

Group Size 3–7

Materials Compact disc or cassette tape player
Compact discs or tapes

Directions Choose a leader. Have participants sit in circle or in line to observe the leader and copy any movements the leader makes. This activity it similar to *"Simon Says"* without the words. Play music to enhance movement. Start slow and simple, working into more complex!

1. Set participants up for comfort—enough room to move freely and observe the leader.
2. Start with moving the head and neck—circles and nods.
3. Move the shoulders—shrugs and in circles, forward and back.
4. Move fingers—playing the piano.
5. Move the arms—out at sides in circles, up and down in front of body.
6. Scoot to the front of the chair and move the trunk—bend forward, lean back.
7. Move the legs—marching, extend legs in front of body and see how long they can be held, flex and extend feet.

Therapeutic Goals

1. To increase or maintain range of motion in upper extremities.
2. To increase or maintain strength and coordination in upper extremities.
3. To increase or maintain range of motion in lower extremities.
4. To increase or maintain strength and coordination in lower extremities.
5. To increase or maintain ability to follow directions.
6. To increase or maintain ability to attend to the task.
7. To increase or maintain ability to complete the task.
8. To increase or maintain strength and endurance.

Contraindications Sensitivity to noise

Comments and Observations

Wishing Well

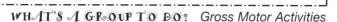

Required Function Levels
Cognitive: 3–2
Sensorimotor: 3–2
Interpersonal: 3–2

Group Size 3–10

Materials Masking tape or yardstick
Buttons in a variety of sizes and colors

Directions Have participants stand or sit in wheelchairs at the line. Each player pitches 5 buttons, one at a time, at the wall. The goal is to see who can land a button closest to the wall. Have each participant choose buttons all of one color for easy identification.

1. At 3 feet from the wall, make a line with the tape or yardstick (parallel to the wall).
2. Line up each person behind the line.
3. Give each participant 5 buttons.
4. Have each person approach the line and take a turn.
5. Have participants toss their buttons against wall so they will fall on the floor.
6. The purpose of the game is to get the button(s) closest to the wall.
7. After each round, the person with the button closest to the wall picks up one button from each player, in addition to their own.
8. Continue the game until one person has all the buttons or the session time has ended.

Therapeutic Goals

1. To increase or maintain range of motion.
2. To increase or maintain strength and coordination in upper extremities.
3. To increase or maintain strength and endurance.
4. To increase or maintain balance.
5. To increase or maintain ability to attend to the task.
6. To increase or maintain ability to follow directions.
7. To improve or maintain proprioception awareness.
8. To increase or maintain ability to complete the task.
9. To increase or maintain fine motor skills.

Comments and Observations

Crazy Walk

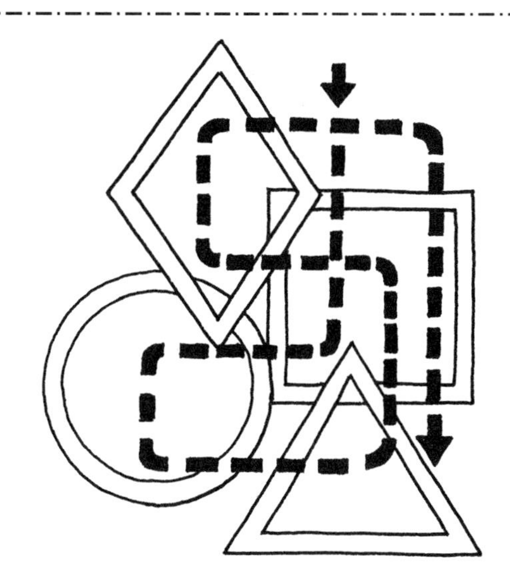

Required Function Levels

Cognitive: 3–2
Sensorimotor: 3–2
Interpersonal: 3–2

Group Size 3–5

Materials

Masking tape for inside maze
Sidewalk chalk for outside maze
Compact disc or tape player
Music on compact discs or tapes

Directions

Participants will walk or use wheelchairs to go through the maze. There will be shapes in the maze that indicate which exercise participants are to stop and perform (e.g., in the triangle everyone snaps their fingers, in the circle everyone moves their arms in circles, in the square everyone marches in place, or in the diamond everyone claps their hands).

1. Tape or chalk a maze for participants to follow (wide enough for wheelchairs). Include a variety of large shapes that will accommodate participants.
2. Start participants moving through the maze.
3. When participants arrive at a shape, have them gather inside it and do activity.
4. Continue through maze and shapes with variety of activities.

Therapeutic Goals

1. To increase or maintain range of motion.
2. To increase or maintain strength and coordination in upper extremities.
3. To increase or maintain strength and endurance.
4. To increase or maintain balance.
5. To increase or maintain ability to attend to the task.
6. To increase or maintain ability to complete the task.
7. To increase or maintain ability to follow directions.
8. To increase or maintain visual perception/discrimination.
9. To increase or maintain strength and coordination in lower extremities.
10. To increase or maintain fine motor skills.

Contraindications Sensitivity to noise

Variations

* Have bottles of bubbles to blow for oral motor skills.
* If the space isn't very large, have participants go through the maze in twos or threes.
* Have participants go through the maze again and do more complex or different movements than the previous round for each shape.
* Jump rope or use paddle balls in one of the spaces.

Comments and Observations

Felicia Norman/ISBN 0761634002/1-800-228-0752/This page is reproducible

Ladybug, Ladybug Fly Away

Required Function Levels

Cognitive: 3–2
Sensorimotor: 3–2
Interpersonal: 3–2

Group Size 3–8

Materials

Cardboard
String (preferably nylon)
Crayons, water-based markers, or poster paints
Oval template
Scissors
Hole punch

Directions

1. Have participants take turns using the 2" oval template to trace a ladybug body on cardboard.
2. Cut the ladybug body out of the cardboard.
3. Have each participant decorate his or her ladybug.
4. Punch a hole or have each participant punch a hole in his or her ladybug's head and thread a 36" length of string through it.
5. Tie one end of the string to a table leg or tape it securely to the wall about 12" from the floor.
6. Have participants start with the ladybug close to their fingers.
7. Pull string taut and bug will twirl around the string.
8. Release the string and the ladybug should slide forward.
9. Keep repeating these actions until someone's ladybug reaches the end of the string, then you have a winner!

Therapeutic Goals

1. To increase or maintain range of motion.
2. To increase or maintain strength and coordination in upper extremities.
3. To increase or maintain strength and endurance.
4. To increase or maintain ability to attend to the task.
5. To increase or maintain ability to complete the task.
6. To increase or maintain ability to follow directions.
7. To increase or maintain fine motor skills.

Comments and Observations

Cognitive Activities

What's Up Doc?

Name That Picture

Animal Caravan

Peanut Butter Bird Snacks

Stringing the Birds Along

Smells Delightful

Mung Growth

Alfalfa Cotton

Baby Birds

Note: In choosing activities from the following section, it is important that you consider age, safety awareness, and appropriateness of an activity based on each participant's evaluated function level. As the leader of the group, you are responsible for ensuring that all health and safety precautions are followed during the group activity.

Sample Measurable Objectives for Cognitive Activities

Goal: To increase or maintain ability to attend to the task.
Objective: Patient will attend to activity for *(specify length of time).*
Objective: Patient will attend to group for *(specify length of time).*

Goal: To improve socialization skills.
Objective: Patient will be able to work on the activity without disrupting others in a group.
Objective: Patient will work cooperatively on the activity with another patient or others.

Goal: To improve or maintain receptive communication skills.
Objective: Patient will be able to follow a simple demonstration.
Objective: Patient will be able to follow one-step oral directions.
Objective: Patient will be able to follow multi-step oral directions.

Goal: To improve or maintain expressive communication skills.
Objective: Patient will use gestures to indicate needs.
Objective: Patient will orally express needs using single words.
Objective: Patient will use phrases or sentences to express needs.

Goal: To increase or maintain ability to follow directions.
Objective: Patient will be able to follow demonstration.
Objective: Patient will be able to follow one-step oral directions.
Objective: Patient will be able to follow multi-step oral directions.

Goal: To improve word retrieval.
Objective: Patient will be able to recall word with picture cues.
Objective: Patient will be able to recall word with verbal cues.

What's Up, Doc?

Required Function Levels

Cognitive: 3–2
Sensorimotor: 3–2
Interpersonal: 3–2

Group Size 3–6

Materials

6 unlike objects
6 similar objects

Directions

Have participants take turns removing an item from the table while one person is looking away. When the other person turns around to the table, ask which item is missing. Start by placing 6 unlike objects (e.g., comb, spoon, pencil, matchbook, coin, slipper) on table. After everyone has successfully attempted guessing, try repeating the game with similar items (e.g., 6 ADL items, 6 kitchen items, items that are same size or color).

1. Place 6 objects on the table.
2. Review the objects with participants.
3. Have one participant turn away while the leader or another participant removes an object from the table.
4. If the participant guesses correctly, return the item to the table.
5. If the participant does not guess correctly, have someone else give the cues.
6. The participant who guessed correctly now gets a turn to remove an item.
7. Go all the way around the table, giving everyone a chance to participate.

Therapeutic Goals

1. To increase or maintain ability to attend to the task.
2. To increase or maintain ability to complete the task.
3. To increase or maintain ability to follow directions.
4. To improve or maintain receptive communication skills.
5. To improve or maintain expressive communication skills.
6. To improve socialization skills.
7. To increase or maintain range of motion.
8. To increase or maintain strength and coordination in upper extremities.
9. To increase or maintain strength and endurance.

Contraindications

Patients with dementia
Patients with visual impairments

Variations

* To increase difficulty, increase the number of objects on the table.
* Have everyone close their eyes and see who can guess correctly first.
* Instead of taking away an item, add one.

Comments and Observations

Name That Picture

Required Function Levels

Cognitive: 3–2
Sensorimotor: 3–2
Interpersonal: 3–2

Group Size 3–7

Materials Pictures of animals, ADL items, kitchenware, clothing, well-known people, etc.
Words that correspond with pictures

Directions Have participants sit around a table for this activity. You can do this activity 1:1 or with a group. It can be a good activity for people with memory or word recall difficulties. The goal of this activity is to match the correct word with the corresponding picture. To increase the difficulty, place pictures and words face down on the table and have each person take turns uncovering matching pairs.

1. Place pictures and words face up on table.
2. See how many pictures and words participants can match without cues.
3. Turn pictures upside down, while participants are watching.
4. Give one member a word and see if they can place it on the appropriate face down picture.
5. Check to see if the guess was correct.
6. If incorrect, give them another chance to guess before giving another member a turn. If they guessed correctly, move to the next person or give them another word to match.

Therapeutic Goals

1. To improve or maintain recall ability.
2. To improve or maintain memory skills.
3. To improve word finding skills.
4. To improve or maintain problem solving skills.
5. To increase or maintain ability to attend to the task.
6. To increase or maintain ability to complete the task.
7. To increase or maintain ability to follow directions.
8. To improve or maintain receptive communication skills.
9. To improve or maintain expressive communication skills.
10. To increase or maintain range of motion.
11. To increase or maintain strength and coordination in upper extremities.
12. To increase or maintain strength and endurance.

Contraindications Patients with dementia
Patients with visual impairments

Comments and Observations

Animal Caravan

Required Function Levels

Cognitive: 3–2
Sensorimotor: 3–2
Interpersonal: 3–2

Group Size 3–10

Materials *Imagination!*

Directions Have participants sit in a circle with or without a table and make up silly sentences about animals traveling in human vehicles to a specific destination. It can be any type of animal, so you might want to determine what category of animals you want to use—house pets, jungle animals, Arctic animals, small wildlife.

1. Choose someone to be the leader and start by making up a silly sentence. For example, *"A penguin rode a skateboard into the woods."*
2. The next person must choose another animal from the same category with a different form of transportation and destination. For example, *"A polar bear rode a train to the beach."*
3. This continues around the table until everyone has had a chance to participate.
4. Change categories and start again!

Therapeutic Goals

1. To increase or maintain ability to attend to the task.
2. To increase or maintain ability to complete the task.
3. To increase or maintain ability to follow directions.
4. To improve or maintain receptive communication skills.
5. To improve or maintain expressive communication skills.
6. To improve or maintain recall ability.
7. To improve or maintain memory skills.
8. To improve word finding skills.
9. To increase or maintain strength and endurance.

Variations

* Use same mode of transportation for all sentences.
* Use same animal for all sentences.
* Use same destination for all sentences.

Comments and Observations

Peanut Butter Bird Snacks

Required Function Levels

Cognitive: 3–2
Sensorimotor: 3–2
Interpersonal: 3–2

Group Size 3–8

Materials

Peanut butter
Wild bird seed mix
Mixing bowl
Large spoon
Onion bags

Directions

Have participants sit around a table for this activity. Have participants take turns adding and mixing the ingredients in the bowl. The follow-up to this activity is a group discussion of the birds they can see and identify eating the snacks.

1. Have the first person scoop 1 cup of peanut butter into the mixing bowl.
2. Add 2 cups of bird seed mix.
3. Have participants take turns stirring all the seeds into the peanut butter.
4. If the mixture is too runny, add more seeds.
5. After it is completely mixed, spoon the mixture into participants' hands and tell them to form it into balls.
6. Place the peanut butter balls into the onion bag. If there is a window in the activity room from which you can see a tree with a low branch, hang the bag on the branch.

Therapeutic Goals

1. To increase or maintain ability to attend to the task.
2. To increase or maintain ability to follow directions.
3. To improve or maintain proprioception awareness.
4. To provide tactile stimulation.
5. To provide olfactory stimulation.
6. To increase or maintain ability to complete the task.
7. To increase or maintain range of motion.
8. To increase or maintain strength and coordination in upper extremities.
9. To increase or maintain strength and endurance.

Variations

* See *Stringing the Birds Along* on page 49.
* Have participants keep journals on the birds they observe and share their findings with the group.
* Hang a dry erase board on which people can list their observations.

Comments and Observations

Stringing the Birds Along

Required Function Levels

Cognitive: 3–2
Sensorimotor: 3–2
Interpersonal: 3

Group Size 3–8

Materials

Unshelled, unsalted peanuts
Apple peels
Orange peels
Yarn
Large needles
Old hangers

Directions

Have participants create bird snacks. The snacks should not be easily acquired by other critters. Find a tree to hang the treat on outside the activity room so that participants can watch the birds.

1. Cut 10" lengths of yarn or ribbon.
2. Thread needle with yarn and pierce a piece of orange peel.
3. Next thread a peanut on the yarn.
4. Vary pieces of fruit with peanuts until 5" of yarn is left free.
5. Bend the bottom of a hanger so that it becomes a diamond shape.
6. Tie the yarn onto bottom of the hanger.
7. Place the hanger on a tree limb or clothesline.

Therapeutic Goals

1. To increase or maintain ability to attend to the task.
2. To increase or maintain ability to follow directions.
3. To improve or maintain proprioception awareness.
4. To provide tactile stimulation.
5. To provide olfactory stimulation.
6. To increase or maintain ability to complete the task.
7. To increase or maintain range of motion.
8. To increase or maintain strength and coordination in upper extremities.
9. To increase or maintain strength and endurance.
10. To increase or maintain fine motor skills.

Variations

* See *Peanut Butter Bird Snacks* on page 47.
* Have participants keep journals on the birds they observe and share their findings with the group.
* Hang a dry erase board on which people can list their observations.

Comments and Observations

Smells Delightful

Required Function Levels

Cognitive: 3–2
Sensorimotor: 3–2
Interpersonal: 3

Group Size 3–10

Materials

3–12 oranges, depending on the size of the group
Whole cloves (better to buy in bulk than in packages, 2 oz. of cloves should cover a medium-size orange)
Spool of curling ribbon in pastels or holiday colors
Small straight pins

Directions

Have participants sit around a table to make the pomanders. You may need to help participants anchor the ribbons to the oranges with small straight pins.

1. Distribute oranges to group members, one per person.
2. Tie ribbon around orange so it can be hung in closet or from curtain rod. It may need to be anchored to the orange with a straight pin.
3. Have each person insert cloves into his or her orange.
4. Cover entire orange or create a design with the cloves.

Therapeutic Goals

1. To increase or maintain ability to attend to the task.
2. To increase or maintain ability to follow directions.
3. To improve or maintain proprioception awareness.
4. To provide tactile stimulation.
5. To provide olfactory stimulation.
6. To increase or maintain ability to complete the task.
7. To increase or maintain range of motion.
8. To increase or maintain strength and coordination in upper extremities.
9. To increase or maintain strength and endurance.
10. To increase or maintain fine motor skills.

Comments and Observations

Mung Growth

Required Function Levels

Cognitive: 3–2
Sensorimotor: 3–2
Interpersonal: 3–1

Group Size 3–8

Materials

Mung beans, alfalfa sprouts, lentils
Saucers
Coffee filters
Water
Large plastic measuring cup

Directions Have participants sit around a table to prepare beans and/or lentils. It takes 5 to 7 days to see growth of the mung beans or lentils. You can do this 1:1 or as a group, providing socialization. The sprouts can be eaten in a salad or stir-fried in a dish that the participants can make.

1. Moisten a coffee filter and place it on a saucer.
2. Place a single layer of lentils or beans on the filter and add a little more water. Water should not cover lentils or beans.
3. Place saucer out of the way of direct sunlight and wait 2 to 3 days before checking on growth.

Therapeutic Goals

1. To increase or maintain ability to attend to the task.
2. To increase or maintain ability to complete the task.
3. To increase or maintain ability to follow directions.
4. To improve or maintain receptive communication skills.
5. To improve or maintain expressive communication skills.
6. To encourage planning skills for grocery shopping.
7. To increase or maintain strength and coordination in upper extremities.
8. To increase or maintain strength and endurance.

Variations

* See *Alfalfa Cotton* on page 55.
* See *Baby Birds* on page 57.
* Split group in half and have one group grow lentils and the other mung beans. Compare the taste of each and the amount of time it took to grow.

Comments and Observations

Alfalfa Cotton

Required Function Levels

Cognitive: 3–2
Sensorimotor: 3–2
Interpersonal: 3–1

Group Size 3–8

Materials Dried alfalfa sprouts
Cotton balls
Baby food jars

Directions Participants will grow alfalfa sprouts over a 4 to 6 day period. Allow them to take their jars back to their rooms and watch the sprouts grow; or you can label each jar and keep them in a cupboard in the group activity room or in a place out of the way of direct sunlight.

1. Place one teaspoon of alfalfa sprouts in each baby food jar.
2. Fill the baby food jar half full with water.
3. Place cotton balls in the jar, on top of the sprouts.
4. Put the jar in a place out of the way of direct sunlight.
5. Check growth in 3 to 4 days.

Therapeutic Goals

1. To increase or maintain ability to attend to the task.
2. To increase or maintain ability to complete the task.
3. To increase or maintain ability to follow directions.
4. To improve or maintain receptive communication skills.
5. To improve or maintain expressive communication skills.
6. To improve and encourage planning skills for grocery shopping.
7. To increase or maintain strength and coordination in upper extremities.
8. To increase or maintain strength and endurance.

Variations

* See *Mung Growth* on page 53.
* See *Baby Birds* on page 57.

Comments and Observations

Baby Birds

Required Function Levels

Cognitive: 3–2
Sensorimotor: 3–2
Interpersonal: 3–1

Group Size 3–8

Materials

3 Tbsp. bird seed per jar
Paper towels
Rubber bands
Narrow glass jars (small horseradish, mustard, or relish jars work well)
Yellow acrylic paint
Water

Directions

Participants will grow bird seed over a 5 to 7 day period. Allow them to take the jars back to their rooms and watch the "baby birds" grow.

1. Paint bird legs on jar and set aside to dry.
2. Place the bird seed in the middle of the paper towel.
3. Bring the four corners of the towel together.
4. Use a rubber band to secure bird seed in middle of towel.
5. Trim the ends of the paper towel so it will fit into the jar.
6. Fill the jar with water.
7. Place the ball of bird seed on top of the jar with the loose ends of paper towel pushed inside the jar.
8. Set the jar in place out of the way of direct sunlight.

Therapeutic Goals

1. To increase or maintain ability to attend to the task.
2. To increase or maintain ability to complete the task.
3. To increase or maintain ability to follow directions.
4. To improve or maintain receptive communication skills.
5. To improve or maintain expressive communication skills.
6. To improve or encourage planning skills for grocery shopping.
7. To increase or maintain strength and coordination in upper extremities.
8. To increase or maintain strength and endurance.
9. To provide tactile stimulation.
10. To increase or maintain fine motor skills.

Variations

* See *Mung Growth* on page 53.
* See *Alfalfa Cotton* on page 55.

Comments and Observations

GAMES

Hot Potato

Paper Clip Relay

Sound Bingo

Chopstick Popcorn Race

Simon Says

Tree, Flower, or Bird?

Song Game

Guess What It Is

Note: In choosing activities from the following section, it is important that you consider age, safety awareness, and appropriateness of an activity based on each participant's evaluated function level. As the leader of the group, you are responsible for ensuring that all health and safety precautions are followed during the group activity.

Sample Measurable Objectives for Games

Goal: To increase or maintain range of motion.

Objective: Patients' range of motion in *(specify upper extremity joint[s])* will be maintained or increased *(specify degrees or within functional limits).*

Goal: To increase or maintain strength and endurance.

Objective: Patient will increase or maintain overall muscle strength and endurance.

Objective: Patient will increase or maintain muscle strength and endurance in *(specify specific muscle group[s] or extremities).*

Goal: To increase or maintain balance.

Objective: Patient will increase or maintain ability to stand *(specify length of time)* without an assistive device.

Goal: To increase or maintain ability to attend to the task.

Objective: Patient will attend to the activity for *(specify length of time).*

Objective: Patient will attend to the group for *(specify length of time).*

Goal: To increase or maintain fine motor skills.

Objective: Patient will demonstrate fine motor dexterity *(specify unilateral or bilateral).*

Goal: To improve or maintain receptive communication skills.

Objective: Patient will be able to follow a simple demonstration.

Objective: Patient will be able to follow one-step oral directions.

Objective: Patient will be able to follow multi-step oral directions.

Goal: To increase or maintain ability to follow directions.

Objective: Patient will be able to follow one-step oral directions.

Objective: Patient will be able to follow multi-step oral directions.

Hot Potato

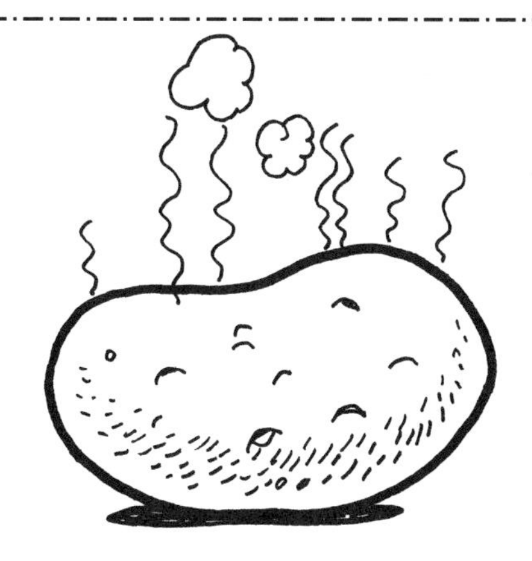

Required Function Levels

Cognitive: 3–2
Sensorimotor: 3–2
Interpersonal: 3–1

Group Size 5–10

Materials

Bean bags to use as *hot potatoes*
Tape player
Tape
Hawaiian leis or scarves

Directions

Participants are seated or standing in circle ready to catch and throw the *hot potato* to other members of the group. Need source of music to be controlled by a *leader* to regulate start and stop. The person holding the *hot potato* is eliminated from winning by donning a Hawaiian lei or something bright. They will still be included in the game but will not be the winner.

1. Toss the *potato* to one participant.
2. Turn the music on.
3. Let participants toss the *potato* around the circle to each other.
4. Turn the music off and see who is caught with the *potato.* The person with the *potato* must wear a lei or scarf.
5. Start the game again.

Therapeutic Goals

1. To increase or maintain range of motion.
2. To increase or maintain strength.
3. To increase or maintain endurance.
4. To increase or maintain balance.
5. To increase or maintain ability to attend to the task.
6. To increase or maintain ability to complete the task.
7. To increase or maintain proprioceptive awareness.

Variations

* Have participants toss the bean bag to each other, calling the name of the person who will receive the *hot potato.* Calling the person's name should help with memory.
* All participants can clap their hands to a slow beat or to music during the activity.

Comments and Observations

Paper Clip Relay

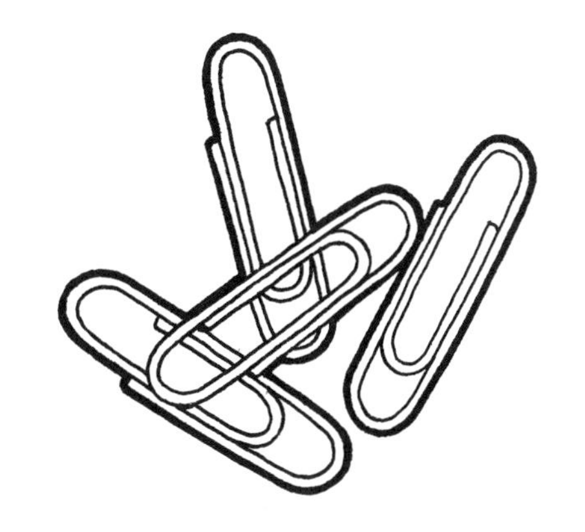

Required Function Levels
Cognitive: 3–2
Sensorimotor: 3–2
Interpersonal: 3–1

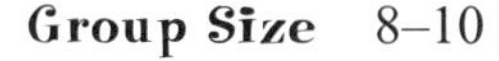

Group Size 8–10

Materials Large paper clips

Directions Have participants stand or sit in two single lines, facing each other. You should have an equal number of participants to divide the group equally. The object of the game is to see which group can pass the paper clips down the line connecting their clip to the chain the fastest.

1. Give the first person in each line two paper clips, give the other members one clip each.
2. The first person connects two clips and passes it to next person.
3. Each person connects his or her clip and passes it down the line.
4. When chain reaches end of line, the person needs to shout or stand up.

Therapeutic Goals

1. To increase or maintain range of motion.
2. To increase or maintain strength.
3. To increase or maintain endurance.
4. To increase or maintain balance.
5. To increase or maintain ability to attend to the task.
6. To increase or maintain ability to complete the task.
7. To increase or maintain proprioceptive awareness.
8. To increase or maintain fine motor skills.
9. To increase or maintain hand–eye coordination.

Variations

* Use small paper clips.
* Try this activity with participants blindfolded.
* Try this activity with participants wearing gloves.
* Vary the activity by passing the chain back up the line with each person removing a clip.
* Have opposite-sided CVA patients team up—right to left and left to right.

Comments and Observations

Sound Bingo

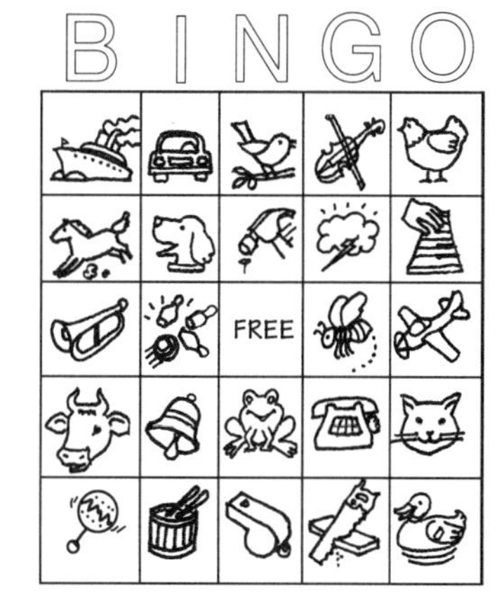

Required Function Levels
Cognitive: 3–2
Sensorimotor: 3–2
Interpersonal: 3–2

Group Size 3–10

Materials Picture Bingo cards (See example on page 105 in the Appendix.)
Plastic chips to cover pictures
Tape player
Tape with sounds that correspond with the Picture Bingo cards

Directions Have the participants listen to the sounds from the tape. Tell them to place a chip on the corresponding picture if it is located on the card in front of them. The first player to cover the designated squares shouts "BINGO!" and wins the game. *You will need to prepare a tape with sound effects for this game. A sample bingo card is included on page 105 in the Appendix.*

1. Tell the players that the first person to cover the squares that match the sounds is the winner. You decide if the players need to match sounds across, down, diagonally, or have a full card to have a bingo.
2. Play the taped sound only once. Wait a reasonable amount of time (this may vary from group to group) before you play the next taped sound.
3. Players should place chips on the pictures that match the sounds.
4. Repeat steps 2 and 3 until a player yells BINGO! Make sure all spaces are correctly covered.
5. Have the winner recite the pictures back to make sure they are correct.

Therapeutic Goals

1. To increase or maintain range of motion.
2. To increase or maintain strength.
3. To increase or maintain endurance.
4. To increase or maintain ability to attend to the task.
5. To increase or maintain ability to complete the task.
6. To enhance auditory stimulation and discrimination.
7. To increase or maintain fine motor skills.
8. To enhance visual scanning.
9. To increase vocalization.

Variations Player can call back sounds instead of names when reciting for "BINGO."

Comments and Observations

Chopstick Popcorn Race

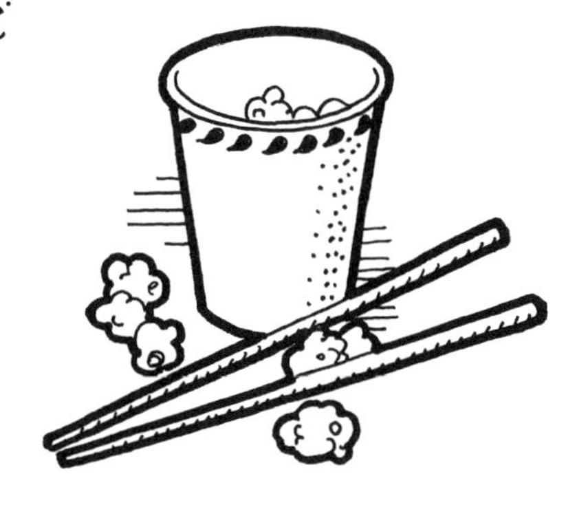

Required Function Levels

Cognitive: 3–2
Sensorimotor: 3–2
Interpersonal: 3–2

Group Size 3–10

Materials

Paper cups
Popcorn
Chopsticks for each player

Directions

Have participants use chopsticks to pick up popcorn from the table to place in cups in front of them. There can be as many participants as can be comfortably seated around the table.

1. Each participant needs to determine most comfortable way to hold chopsticks.
2. Set a cup in front of each player.
3. Place large piles of popcorn on the table in strategic places.
4. Start by saying, "Get set, GO!" Participants must use chopsticks to place as much popcorn as they can in their cups.
5. The first person with a full cup must stand up or shout "full" and is the winner.

Therapeutic Goals

1. To increase or maintain range of motion.
2. To increase or maintain strength.
3. To increase or maintain endurance.
4. To increase or maintain ability to attend to the task.
5. To increase or maintain ability to complete the task.
6. To increase or maintain proprioceptive awareness.
7. To increase or maintain fine motor skills.
8. To increase or maintain hand–eye coordination.

Variations

* Use one hand only or try a spoon instead of chopsticks.
* To improve facial muscle and lung capacity use straws (various *lengths and widths*) with cheese puffs or cotton balls.
* You might have to adhere the cups to the table surface to make it less confusing and difficult.

Comments and Observations

Simon Says

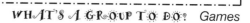

Required Function Levels

Cognitive: 3–2
Sensorimotor: 3–2
Interpersonal: 3–1

Group Size As many people as you can have comfortably in the room, seated an arm's length apart

Materials Chairs
Hawaiian leis or scarves

Directions "Simon" commands participants to follow physical motions. If participants respond to commands not preceded by "Simon says" they must wear a lei and sit out of the game. The person (or people) who responds appropriately throughout the game is the winner.

1. Have Simon command participants to engage in activities and demonstrate them, such as, "Simon says, 'touch your knees' or 'Put your hands on your head.'"
2. Participants should respond to Simon's commands.
3. Give leis to participants who respond incorrectly and remind them that they are not to participate in the remainder of the game.

Therapeutic Goals

1. To increase or maintain range of motion.
2. To increase or maintain strength and endurance.
3. To increase or maintain balance.
4. To increase or maintain ability to attend to the task.
5. To increase or maintain ability to complete the task.
6. To increase or maintain proprioceptive awareness.
7. To increase or maintain fine motor skills.
8. To improve or maintain ability to follow directions.
9. To improve or maintain receptive communication.

Contraindications If there is too much chatting among the group, people with hearing impairments may find it difficult to understand Simon's directions.

Comments and Observations

Tree, Flower, or Bird?

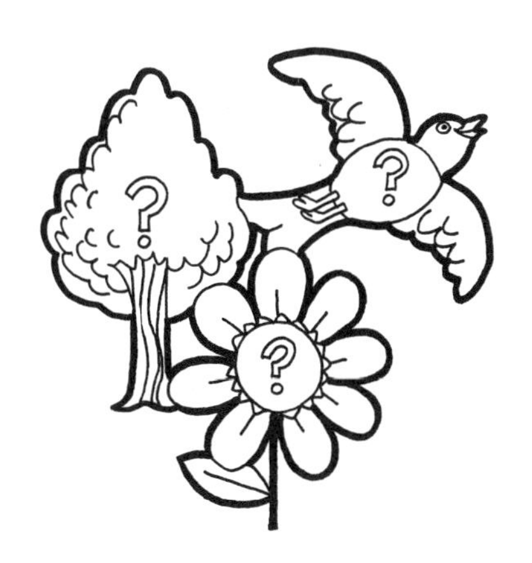

Required Function Levels

Cognitive: 3–2
Sensorimotor: 3–2
Interpersonal: 3–1

Group Size 5 or more

Materials None

Directions Have participants sit in a circle and select one person to be the leader and to start. Explain to participants that the object is *not* to be in the center. Brainstorm with entire group to come up with lists of each: trees, flowers, and birds. This will stimulate the participants. If participants need to, they can look and then mark off ones used because the names *can only be used once—answers cannot be repeated.*

1. The leader sits in the middle of the circle and begins by saying, "Tree, Flower, or Bird?—Tree" and points to a member of the circle.
2. The player must think of a name before the leader counts to 10.
3. If the player succeeds in naming a tree before the leader counts to 10, then the leader must stay in the middle of the circle and point to another player.
4. The leader repeats this process until a player can't think of a name before the leader counts to 10. When a player can't think of a name, he or she must switch places with the leader.

Therapeutic Goals

1. To increase or maintain ability to attend to the task.
2. To improve or maintain receptive communication.
3. To improve or maintain expressive communication.
4. To enhance recall ability.
5. To improve or maintain ability to follow directions.
6. To improve or maintain gross motor skills.
7. To improve or maintain range of motion.

Comments and Observations

Song Game

Required Function Levels

Cognitive: 3–2
Sensorimotor: 3–1
Interpersonal: 3–2

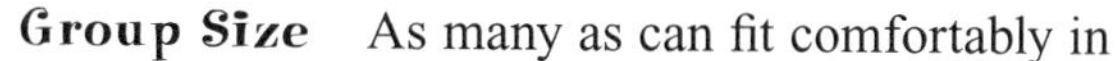

Group Size As many as can fit comfortably in the room

Materials Topic Cards (3" x 5" index cards are a good size to use)
Buzzer or whistle
Chairs
Pad and pencil or chalkboard and chalk

Directions The object of this game is to sing a line of song lyrics that incorporate the word on a given Topic Card. The team or person who correctly sings the lyrics, which must be at least eight words, earns one point. You can continue the game for 15 to 45 minutes, depending on the group's interest. The team with the most points wins.

1. Select a conductor. The conductor shuffles the Topic Cards and chooses a card from the top of the deck. The conductor reads aloud the word on the card to the teams or players, keeps score, and must pay attention to who is the first player to raise his or her hand.
2. Once the topic word has been read, the conductor calls on a team or person who must try to score points by successfully singing eight or more words of a song that includes the topic word. For example, if the topic word is roll, someone may come up with song lyrics about rock and *roll.*
3. Each person must raise his or her hand and be recognized before singing.
4. If the game is played in teams, each team must choose a team member to respond/sing the answer. No other team members may respond while someone is singing.
5. The player called on must respond within 1 minute or 1 point is awarded to the other team or other players.

Therapeutic Goals

1. To increase or maintain ability to attend to the task.
2. To improve or maintain receptive communication.
3. To improve or maintain expressive communication.
4. To enhance recall ability.
5. To improve or maintain ability to follow directions.

Variations

* Song can include all varieties of music.
* Player may consider the topic word with different endings, i.e., *-ly, -ing, -ed.*
* Try this activity at holiday times with holiday songs.

Comments and Observations

Guess What it is

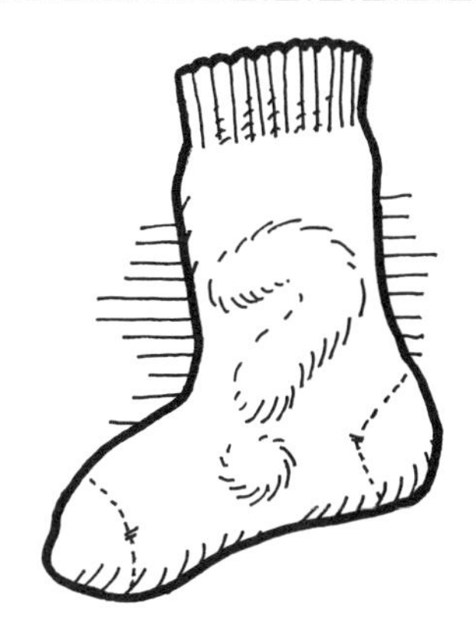

Required Function Levels

Cognitive: 3–2
Sensorimotor: 3–2
Interpersonal: 3–2

Group Size As many as can fit comfortably in the room

Materials
Chairs
Items to be hidden
One sock for each item
Masking tape to number the items
Timer
Answer key (You will need to create this based on the items you have.)
Answer sheets

Directions The goal is to correctly identify the items hidden in the socks. This can be done with hands or with feet (wearing socks) for more of a challenge. The items can be classified into things you find in the kitchen (e.g., measuring spoons, cake decorator, wooden spoon, spatula), bathroom items, or items from any other area in the home.

1. State where items hidden can be found in the house.
2. Pass out answer sheets.
3. If participants are using their feet, have them remove their shoes, but not their socks.
4. Pass out an item to each person. (If they are using feet, place it at their feet—no hands allowed!)
5. Each participant will be given 1 minute to feel the object and write his or her guess on the Answer Sheet.
6. When time is up, have participants pass the items they have to the right and get ready to guess the next item they've received.
7. After all items have been passed around and everyone has had a chance to guess each item, read aloud the Answer Key to see who guessed the most items correctly!

Therapeutic Goals

1. To increase or maintain ability to attend to the task.
2. To improve or maintain receptive communication.
3. To improve or maintain expressive communication.
4. To enhance recall ability.
5. To improve or maintain ability to follow directions.
6. To improve or maintain fine motor skills.
7. To improve tactile stimulation.
8. To improve or maintain sterognosis.

Comments and Observations

CRAFTS

Country Hat Magnet

Butterfly Magnet

Picture Frame Magnet

Tissue Paper Sun Catcher

Gingerbread Paper Doll

Christmas Poinsettia

Christmas Tree Napkin Ring

Reindeer Magnet

Paper Snowflakes

Candy Heart Pack

Clothespin Easter Bunnies

Note: In choosing activities from the following section, it is important that you consider age, safety awareness, and appropriateness of an activity based on each participant's evaluated function level. As the leader of the group, you are responsible for ensuring that all health and safety precautions are followed during the group activity.

All craft activities are for 3 to 10 participants seated around a table or working surface. Participants should be able to see the group leader/facilitator.

Sample Measurable Objectives for Crafts

Goal: Provide tactile stimulation.
Objective: Patient will be able to identify objects on the basis of touch.
Objective: Patient will discriminate between objects on the basis of texture.

Goal: To increase or maintain fine motor skills.
Objective: Patient will demonstrate fine motor dexterity *(specify unilateral or bilateral).*

Goal: To increase or maintain ability to attend to the task.
Objective: Patient will attend to the activity for *(specify length of time).*
Objective: Patient will attend to the group for *(specify length of time).*

Goal: To increase or maintain ability to follow directions.
Objective: Patient will be able to follow one-step oral directions.
Objective: Patient will be able to follow multi-step oral directions.

Goal: To increase or maintain strength and endurance.
Objective: Patient will increase or maintain upper extremity muscle strength and endurance.
Objective: Patient will increase or maintain hand/finger muscle strength and endurance.

Country Hat Magnet

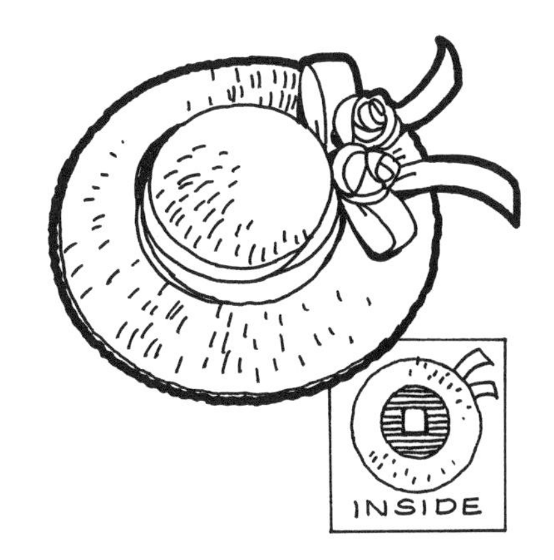

Required Function Levels

Cognitive: 3–2
Sensorimotor: 3–2
Interpersonal: 3–1

Materials

Per person:
1) Miniature straw hat
2) Miniature ribbon roses
1) 9" length of 1/8" wide ribbon
2) 5" lengths of 3/16" wide ribbon
1) Self adhesive magnet
1) 2 1/2" square pieces of construction paper
Scissors
Tacky glue

Directions

1. Using tacky glue, attach both pieces of 3/16" ribbon around the center base of the hat. Ribbons can be partially overlapping or one on top of the other.
2. Tie the 1/8" ribbon into a small bow and trim to the desired length.
3. Use tacky glue to attach the bow to the seam of the 3/16" ribbons already on the hat.
4. Glue both ribbon roses to the center of the bow.
5. Cut a circle out of the construction paper to cover the inside of the hat.
6. Glue the construction paper to the inside of the hat.
7. Attach a self-adhesive magnet to the construction paper mount.

Therapeutic Goals

1. To increase or maintain fine motor skills.
2. To increase or maintain ability to attend to the task.
3. To increase or maintain ability to complete the task.
4. To increase or maintain ability to follow directions.
5. To increase or maintain strength and endurance.
6. To provide tactile stimulation.

Comments and Observations

Butterfly Magnet

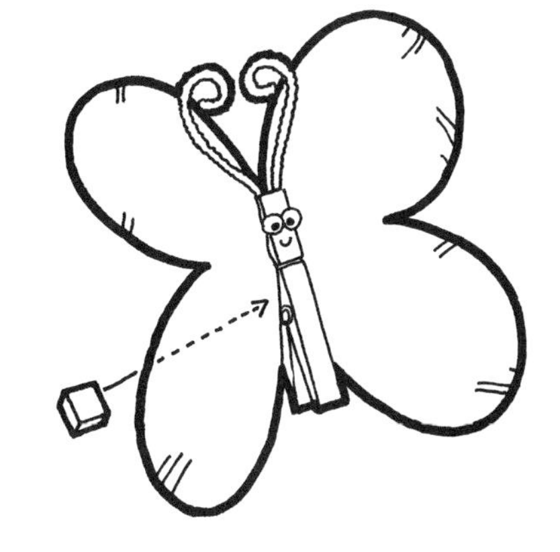

Required Function Levels

Cognitive: 3–2
Sensorimotor: 3–2
Interpersonal: 3–1

Materials

Per person:
1) 6 1/8" x 6 1/8" piece of colored tissue paper
1) pinch clothespin
1) 1" chenille stem
1) self-adhesive magnet
2) 5mm wiggle eyes
Scissors
Tacky glue

Directions

1. Fold the tissue paper in half.
2. Fold it in half again so that it looks like a small square.
3. Making sure the folded side is on the left, cut the bottom right corner and round up to the top right corner.
4. Turn the square so that the folded side is on the right. Cut the right top and bottom corners so that they are rounded.
5. Open the square, turn it over, and put a thin strip of glue on the folded line.
6. Slide the tissue paper into the clothespin so the glue is securing the tissue paper to the clothespin.
7. Glue the eyes to the top part of the clothespin.
8. Secure the self-adhesive magnet to the clothespin.
9. Bend the chenille stem in half. Separate it into a "V" shape and round the ends to look like the tips of antennae.
10. Glue the base of the "V" to the back of the butterfly's head.

Therapeutic Goals

1. To increase or maintain fine motor skills.
2. To increase or maintain ability to attend to the task.
3. To increase or maintain ability to complete the task.
4. To increase or maintain ability to follow directions.
5. To increase or maintain strength and endurance.
6. To provide tactile stimulation.

Comments and Observations

Picture Frame Magnet

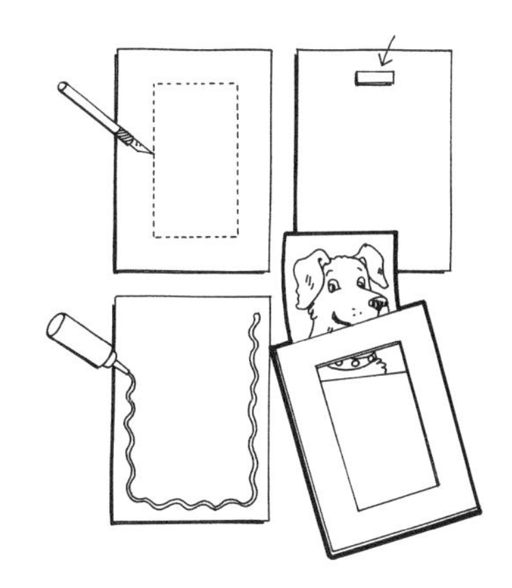

Required Function Levels

Cognitive: 3–2
Sensorimotor: 3–2
Interpersonal: 3–1

Materials

Per person:
2) 5" x 7" pieces of poster board
1) 1" self-adhesive magnet
Scissors or utility knife
Pencils
Tacky glue
Decorations: sequins, glitter, ribbon, buttons, stickers

Directions

1. Take 5" x 7" pieces of poster board and draw a line 1 1/4" in from edge all the way around on one piece. (See diagram on page 104 in the Appendix.)
2. Using scissors, cut out the middle piece; this will leave an opening for a picture when the project is completed.
3. Adhere the magnet to the uncut piece of poster board.
4. Place both pieces of poster board side by side, make sure the magnet side is down.
5. Glue along the edge of the right, left, and bottom sides of the uncut piece. Leave the top unglued in order to put the picture in the frame.
6. Place the front piece (the one with the opening) onto the back piece that has the glue.
7. Now your picture frame is complete! Use decorations to create a personal touch.

Therapeutic Goals

1. To increase or maintain fine motor skills.
2. To increase or maintain ability to attend to the task.
3. To increase or maintain ability to complete the task.
4. To increase or maintain ability to follow directions.
5. To increase or maintain strength and endurance.
6. To provide tactile stimulation.

Comments and Observations

Tissue Paper Sun Catcher

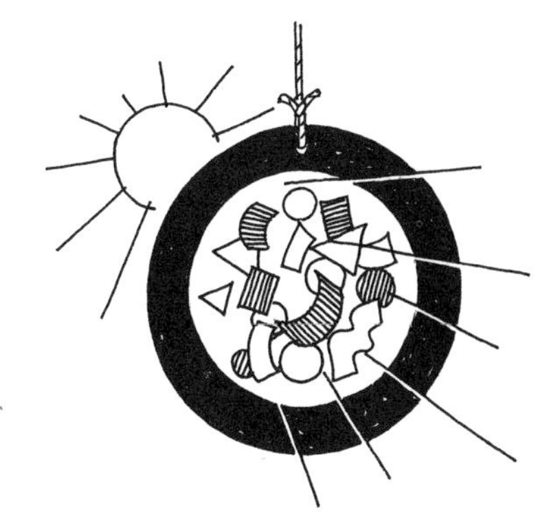

Required Function Levels

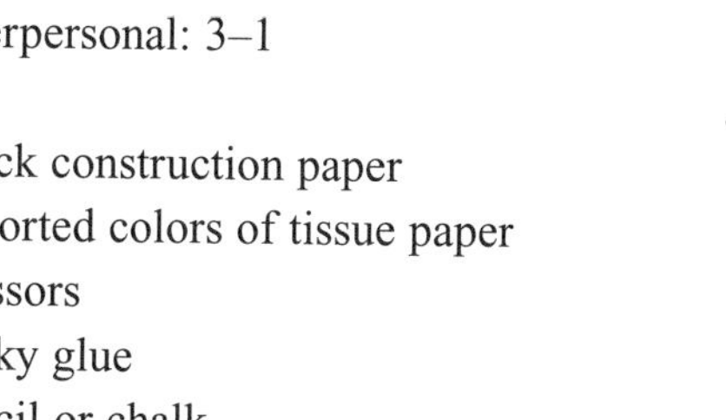

Cognitive: 3–2
Sensorimotor: 3–2
Interpersonal: 3–1

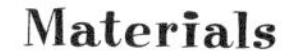

Materials
Black construction paper
Assorted colors of tissue paper
Scissors
Tacky glue
Pencil or chalk

Directions
1. Draw a 6" or 8" circle with 1" width on the black construction paper. After drawing the frame, cut it out.
2. Place the frame on a piece of tissue paper and trace around the *outside* of the frame.
3. Remove the frame and cut out the circle of tissue paper.
4. Using other pieces of tissue paper, cut out small pieces to create design. It's okay if pieces overlap.
5. Spread a thin layer of glue on one side of the frame.
6. Put the frame on top of the tissue paper circle.
7. Press firmly around the frame to make sure it sticks to the tissue paper.

Therapeutic Goals
1. To increase or maintain fine motor skills.
2. To increase or maintain ability to attend to the task.
3. To increase or maintain ability to complete the task.
4. To increase or maintain ability to follow directions.
5. To increase or maintain strength and endurance.
6. To provide tactile stimulation.

Variations
* Use black fabric paint to go over the edges of the tissue paper design.
* Use glitter and sequins to enhance design.

Comments and Observations

Gingerbread Paper Doll

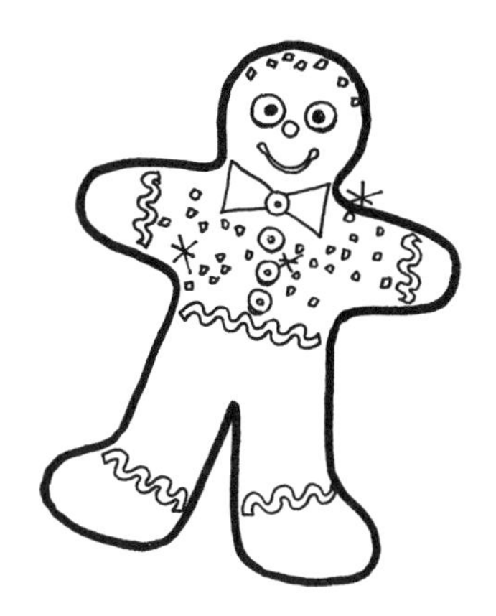

Required Function Levels

Cognitive: 3–2
Sensorimotor: 3–2
Interpersonal: 3–1

Materials

Brown paper bags or a roll of brown butcher paper
Glitter glue
Tacky glue
Ribbons
Buttons
Sequins
Rick-rack
Wiggle eyes
Gingerbread Man pattern (cookie cutter)
Scissors

Directions

1. Make a gingerbread man on brown paper from a pattern.
2. Cut out the gingerbread man.
3. Use various materials to be creative and make a one of a kind gingerbread doll!
4. Use rick-rack to make hands and feet.
5. Use sequins or dots of glitter for buttons.

Therapeutic Goals

1. To increase or maintain fine motor skills.
2. To increase or maintain ability to attend to the task.
3. To increase or maintain ability to complete the task.
4. To increase or maintain ability to follow directions.
5. To increase or maintain strength and endurance.
6. To provide tactile stimulation.

Variations

* Fold the paper to make a string of gingerbread men.
* Use white paper to make snowmen.

Comments and Observations

Christmas Poinsettia

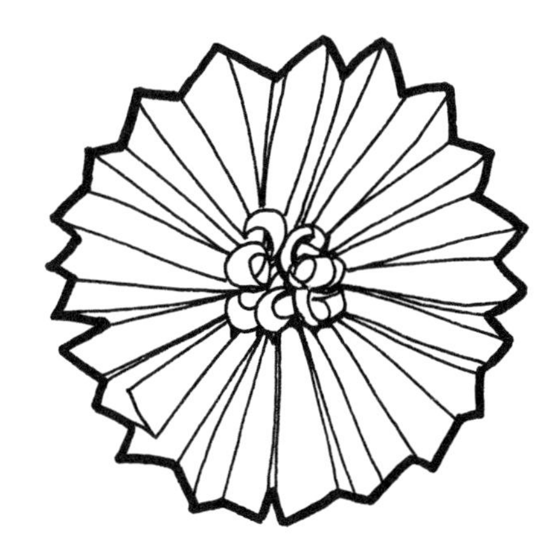

Required Function Levels

Cognitive: 3–2
Sensorimotor: 3–2
Interpersonal: 3–1

Materials

Scissors
9" square red napkins
Twist ties
Curling ribbon, yellow or gold

Directions

1. Open napkin and cut along the folds into 4 pieces of equal size.
2. Line up 4 napkin pieces vertically so that each piece is in diamond shape with the points meeting and overlapping by 1/4".
3. Starting with the napkin closest to you, fold the napkins like a paper fan at center point, working your way up to each piece of napkin.
4. Wrap twist tie around the center point of the napkins and secure tightly.
5. Cut a piece of curling ribbon to tie over the twist tie.
6. Using scissors, use the blunt edge of the scissors and curl the ribbon toward the front of the poinsettia.

Therapeutic Goals

1. To increase or maintain range of motion.
2. To increase or maintain fine motor skills.
3. To increase or maintain strength and endurance.
4. To increase or maintain ability to attend to the task.
5. To increase or maintain ability to complete the task.
6. To increase or maintain ability to follow directions.
7. To provide tactile stimulation.

Comments and Observations

Christmas Tree Napkin Ring

Required Function Levels

Cognitive: 3–2
Sensorimotor: 3–2
Interpersonal: 3–1

Materials

2) Fun Foam™ sheets per participant, 1 green 2" x 2" and 1 red 1" x 5"
Tree pattern
Assorted shape sequins
Gold star sequins
Ribbon
Glitter glue
Scissors
Tacky glue
Clothespins

Directions

To make the napkin ring:

1. Cut a 1" x 5" strip out of the red Fun Foam™.
2. Overlap ends 1/2" and glue.
3. Use a pinch clothespin to clamp the seam together until the glue dries (about 10 minutes).

To make a Christmas tree:

1. Cut out a Christmas tree shape from the green Fun Foam™.
2. Decorate the tree shape with ribbon, sequins, and glitter. Allow the glue to dry before attaching the napkin ring.

Glue the napkin ring along the seam to the back of the tree shape and allow the glue to dry thoroughly.

Therapeutic Goals

1. To increase or maintain range of motion.
2. To increase or maintain fine motor skills.
3. To increase or maintain strength and endurance.
4. To increase or maintain ability to attend to the task.
5. To increase or maintain ability to complete the task.
6. To increase or maintain ability to follow directions.
7. To provide tactile stimulation.

Variations

Use different colors of Fun Foam™ for different occasions or holidays.

Comments and Observations

Reindeer Magnet

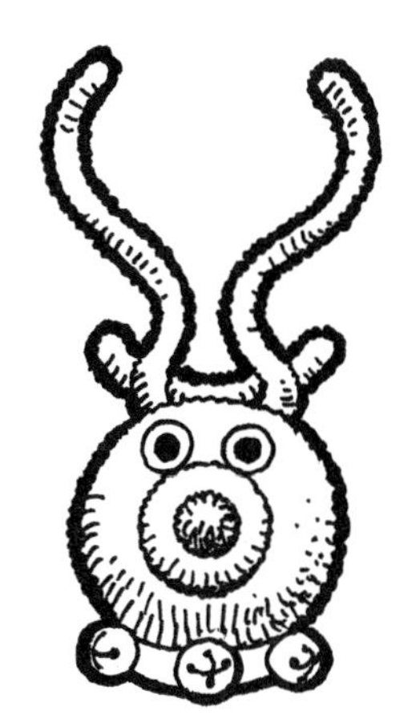

Required Function Levels

Cognitive: 3
Sensorimotor: 3
Interpersonal: 3–1

Materials

Per person:
1) 1" tan pom-pom
1) 1/2" tan pom-pom
1) 7mm red pom-pom
2) 7mm wiggle eyes
1) 1/16" thick craft cork ½" in diameter
2) 1/4" chenille stems
2) 1/2" chenille stems
1) 1/4" ribbon
2) 6mm bells
1) magnet, 1/2" in diameter

Directions

1. Take the tan 1" pom-pom and push away the yarn until you find the middle of it.
2. Glue the cork to the bare spot on the pom-pom.
3. Push away the yarn of the tan 1/2" pom-pom to find the middle of it and glue it to the other side of the 1" pom-pom. (See the diagram on page 109 in the Appendix.)
4. Glue the 7mm red pom-pom to middle of the 1/2" tan pom-pom.
5. Glue eyes above the 1/2" tan pom-pom onto the 1" tan pom-pom.
6. Take the 1/2" chenille stem and bend it into a "U" shape.
7. Take the 1/4" chenille stem and twist it over the "U" shaped stem from step 6.
8. Glue the chenille stems behind the eyes on the top of the 1" tan pom-pom.
9. Glue ribbon to the bottom of the 1" tan pom-pom.
10. Glue the magnet to the back of the cork.

Therapeutic Goals

1. To increase or maintain fine motor skills.
2. To increase or maintain ability to attend to the task.
3. To increase or maintain ability to complete the task.
4. To increase or maintain ability to follow directions.
5. To increase or maintain strength and endurance.
6. To provide tactile stimulation.

Comments and Observations

Paper Snowflakes

Required Function Levels

Cognitive: 3–2
Sensorimotor: 3–2
Interpersonal: 3–1

Materials 8 1/2" x 11" sheets of paper (white typing paper or colored construction paper works)

Directions This is simple as long as paper is folded properly.

1. Fold the paper in half as shown in Diagram A by folding paper in half (along the 8 1/2" edge).
2. Fold the paper in half again as shown in Diagram B by bringing the left half over to the right half.
3. Cut the folded square diagonally, from bottom right to top left corners, making sure not to cut on the folded sides of the square as shown in Diagram C.
4. Now you will cut 3 to 4 small triangles on each of the three sides making sure triangles do not touch as shown in Diagram D.
5. Unfold the snowflake to view your finished product!

Therapeutic Goals

1. To increase or maintain fine motor skills.
2. To increase or maintain ability to attend to the task.
3. To increase or maintain ability to complete the task.
4. To increase or maintain ability to follow directions.
5. To increase or maintain strength and endurance.

Variations Participants can get more intricate with cut-outs, depending on their ability to manipulate scissors and the thickness of the paper.

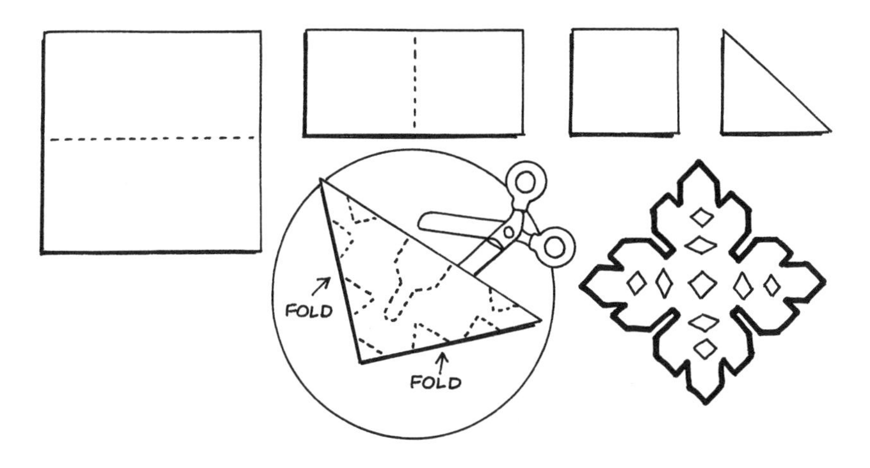

Comments and Observations

Candy Heart Pack

Required Function Levels

Cognitive: 3–2
Sensorimotor: 3–2
Interpersonal: 3–1

Materials

Per person:
6" x 12" piece of clear vinyl
33" of 1/4" ribbon
Small candy pieces
Scissors
Hole punch (1/4")

Directions

1. Fold the vinyl in half, so that the result is a 6" x 6" square.
2. Trace a heart on the vinyl.
3. Cut out the heart. Do not separate the pieces of vinyl.
4. Punch holes all the way around the outside of the heart, about 1/8" away from the edge. Consistent spacing looks nice and is more challenging. (See the diagram on page 111 in the Appendix.)
5. At the bottom of the heart, fold the ribbon in half and start lacing up each side of the heart.
6. When heart is laced up half way, separate the pieces of vinyl.
7. Place pieces of candy in the heart.
8. Finish lacing heart.
9. Tie a bow in the ribbon to close the heart.

Therapeutic Goals

1. To increase or maintain range of motion.
2. To increase or maintain fine motor skills.
3. To increase or maintain ability to attend to the task.
4. To increase or maintain ability to complete the task.
5. To increase or maintain ability to follow directions.
6. To increase or maintain strength and endurance.
7. To provide tactile stimulation.

Variations

* Use fabric or acrylic paints to decorate heart.
* Use 1/8" hole punch and 1/8" ribbon to increase time and fine motor skills.
* Can be used for different occasions or holidays.

Comments and Observations

Clothespin Easter Bunnies

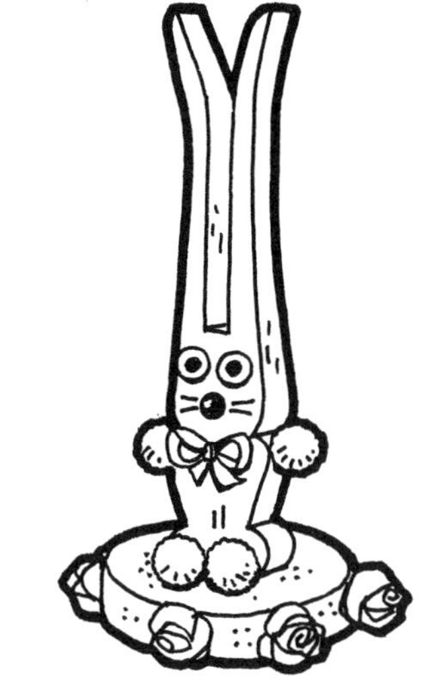

Required Function Levels

Cognitive: 3–2
Sensorimotor: 3–2
Interpersonal: 3–1

Materials

1) Small flat clothespin
4) 5mm tan pom-poms
1) 5mm white pom-pom
2) 4mm wiggle eyes
1) 3mm half-round bead
Spool of 1/8" ribbon
Tacky glue
Fine felt-tipped black marker
Fun Foam™
Small ribbon roses

Directions

1. Glue the eyes on the face of the bunny. (See the diagram on page 113 in the Appendix.)
2. Glue the nose just below the eyes, leaving room for the bow.
3. Draw whiskers from the nose with a felt tip pen.
4. Glue two pom-poms to the bottom front of clothespin for feet.
5. Glue two pom-poms to each side of clothespin, below the face for arms.
6. Use the 1/8" ribbon to wrap around the neck and make a small bow for the front of the bunny.
7. Glue the bow to the front of the bunny, below the nose and above arms.
8. Glue the white pom-pom to the back of the clothespin for the tail.
9. Glue the bottom of the bunny to the foam base.
10. Glue ribbon roses around the base of the bunny.

Therapeutic Goals

1. To increase or maintain fine motor skills.
2. To increase or maintain ability to attend to the task.
3. To increase or maintain ability to follow directions.
4. To increase or maintain strength and endurance.
5. To provide tactile stimulation.
6. To increase or maintain ability to complete the task.

Variations

* Instead of gluing on a tail, use a small strip of magnet.
* Use large clothespins and corresponding larger sizes of materials.

Comments and Observations

Appendix

Lists of Christmas Songs and Nursery Rhymes

Example of a Sound Bingo Card

Picture Frame Magnet Diagram

Reindeer Magnet Diagram

Candy Heart Pack Diagram

Clothespin Easter Bunny Diagram

Christmas Songs

Deck the Halls
Here We Come A-Caroling
Silent Night
Up on the House Top
Away in a Manger
The First Noel
O Come All Ye Faithful
The 12 Days of Christmas
Winter Wonderland
Rudolph, the Red-Nosed Reindeer
Santa Claus is Comin' to Town
Jingle Bells
Frosty the Snowman
O Christmas Tree
God Rest Ye Merry, Gentlemen
O Little Town of Bethlehem
It Came Upon the Midnight Clear
Hark! The Herald Angels Sing
Joy to the World
We Wish You a Merry Christmas

Nursery Rhymes

Old Mother Hubbard
Hey Diddle Diddle
Little Bo Peep
Hickory Dickory Dock
Baa Baa Black Sheep
Jack Be Nimble
Five Little Pigs
Peter, Peter Pumpkin Eater
Humpty Dumpty
Ladybug, Ladybug
24 Blackbirds in a Pie

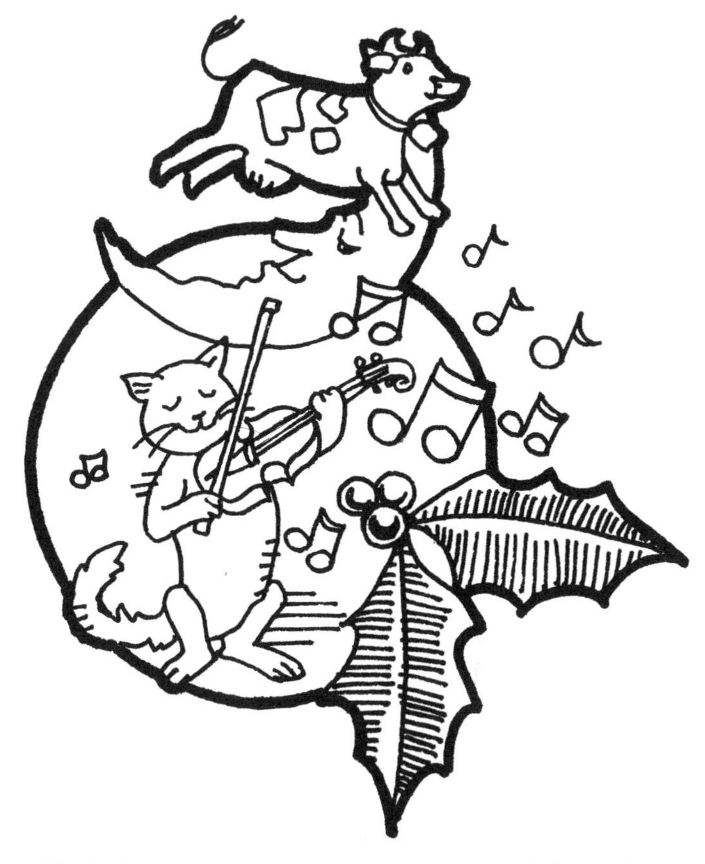

Sound Bingo

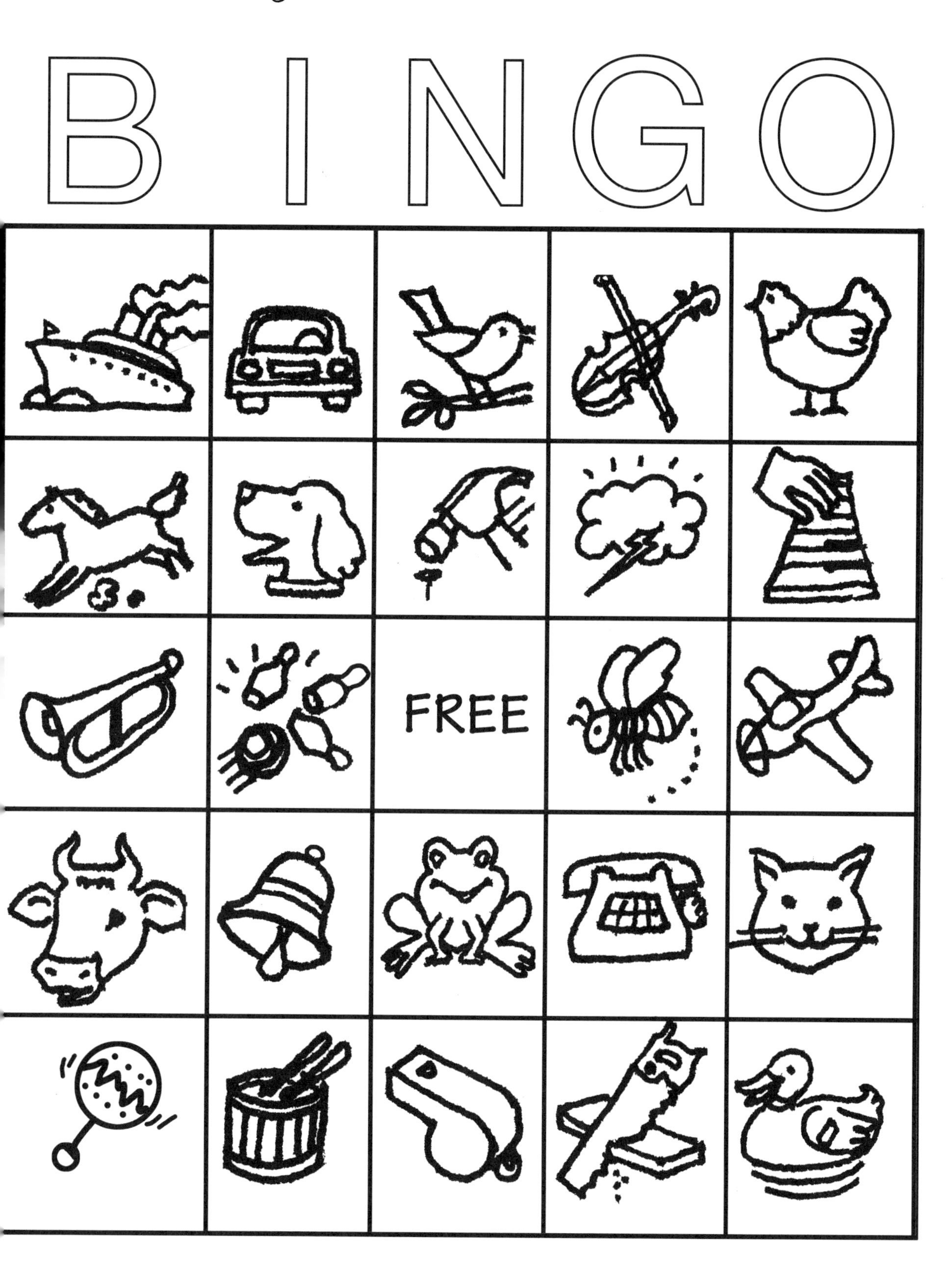

Picture Frame Magnet

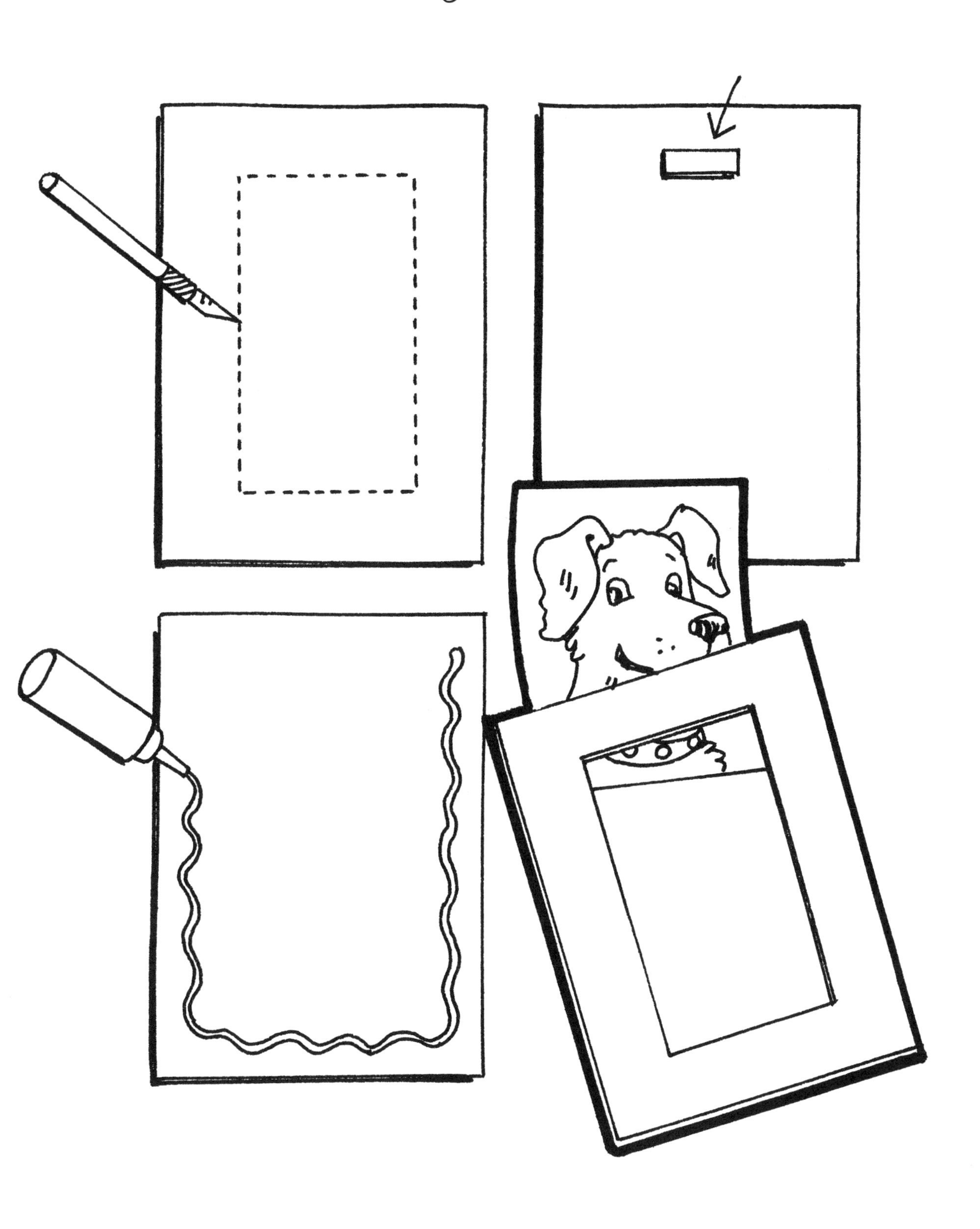

Reindeer Magnet

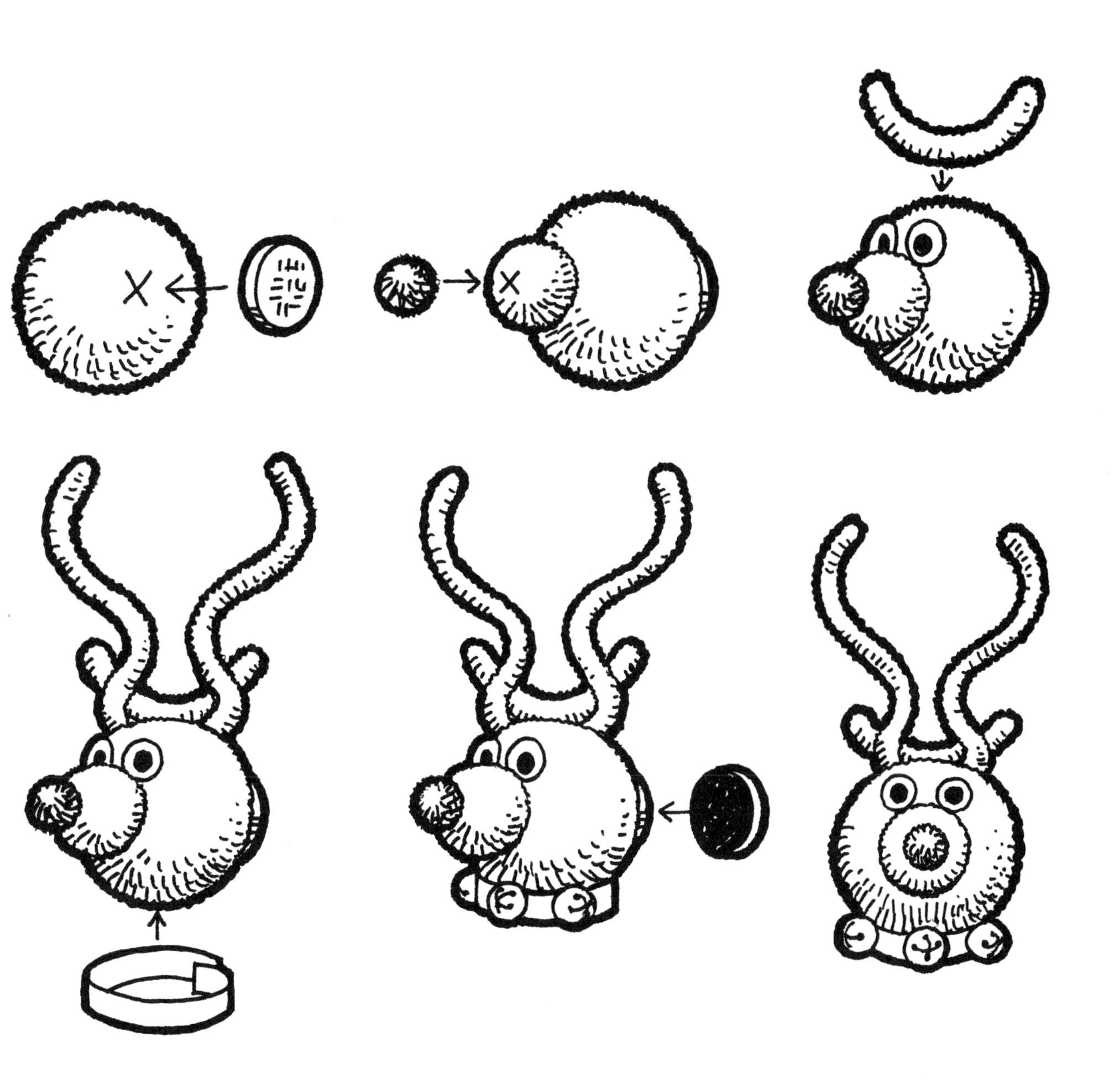

Candy Heart Pack

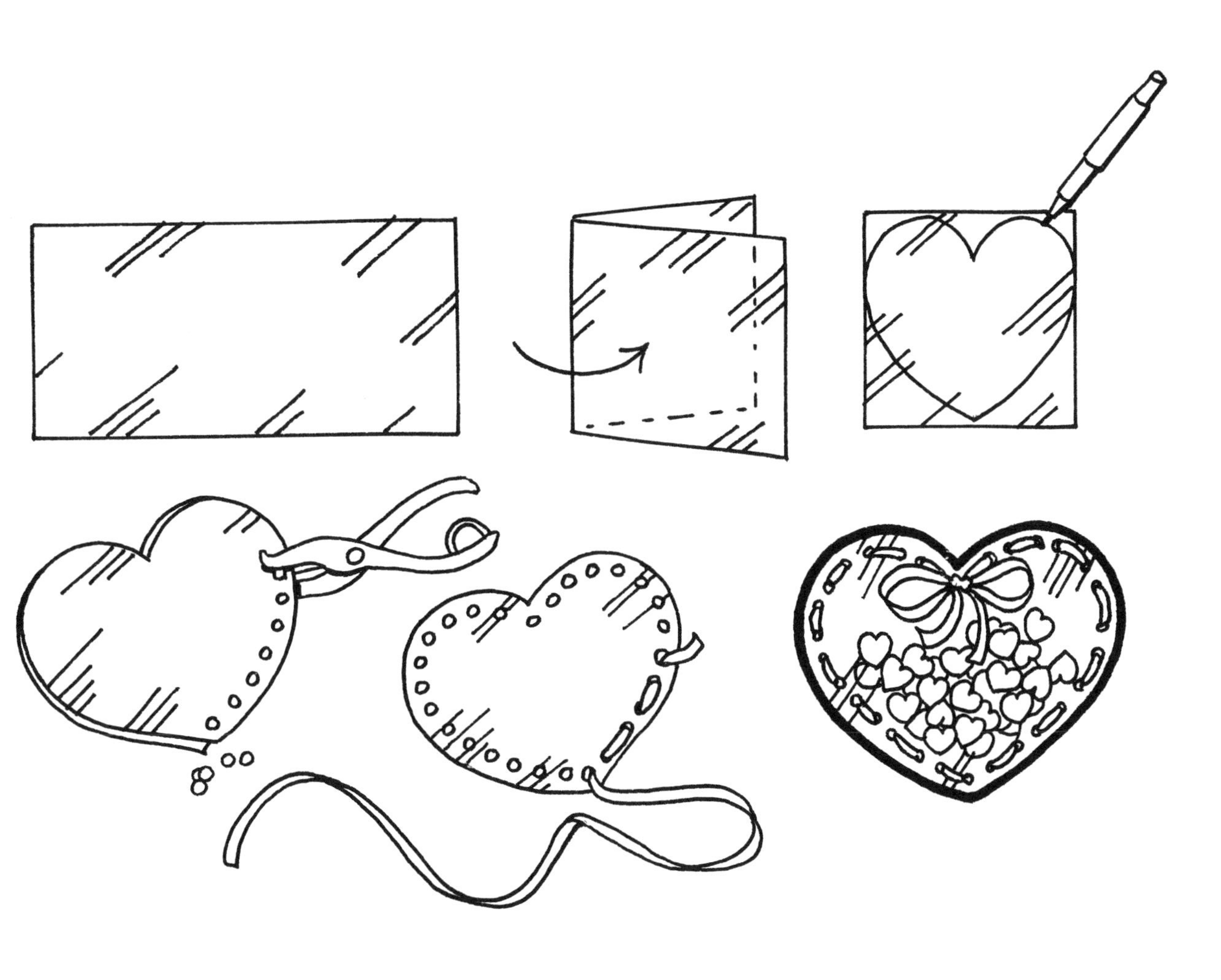

Clothespin Easter Bunnies

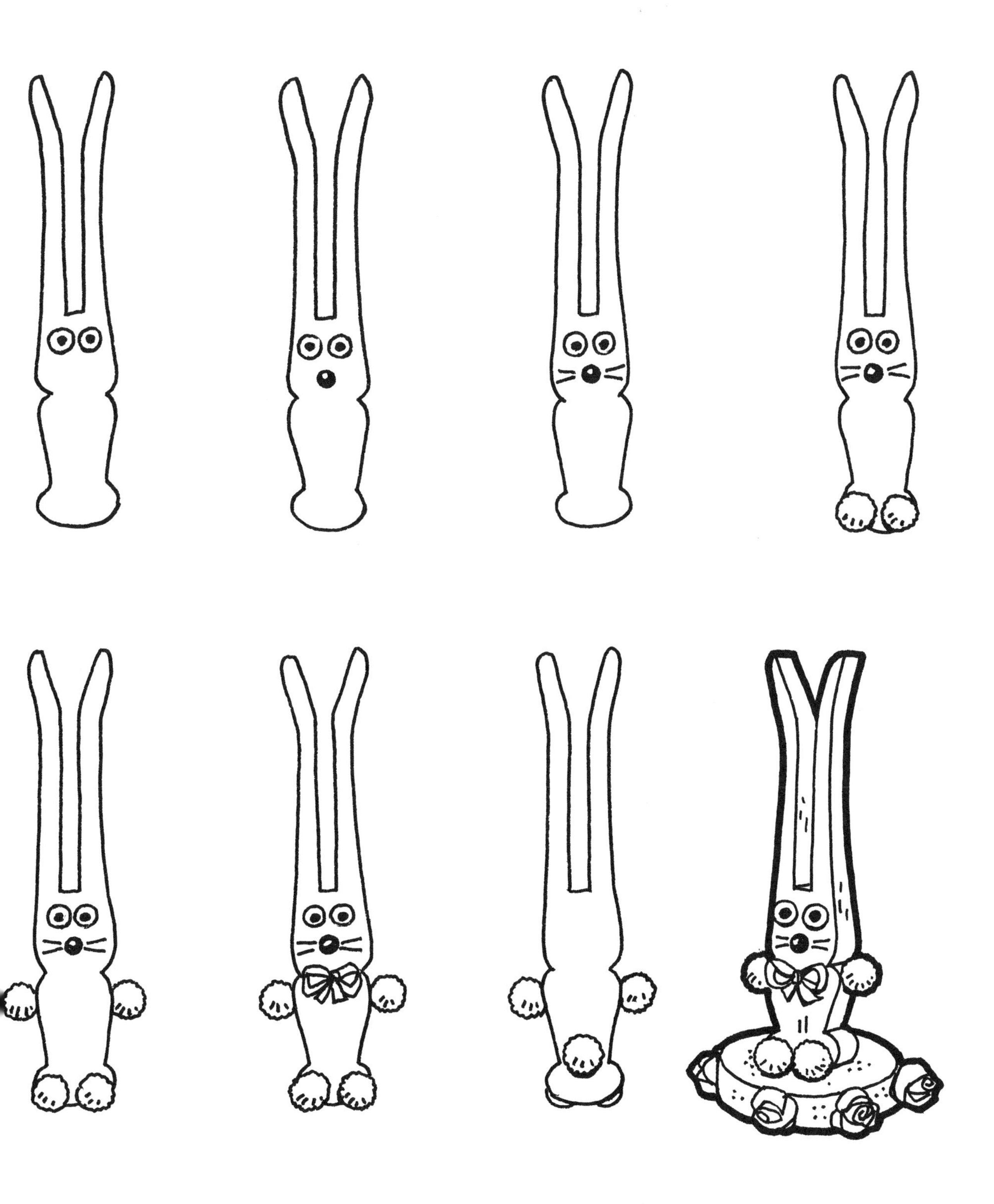

6463 02